THE GERD

AND

ACID REFLUX DIET

COOKBOOK

Mouthwatering, High-Fiber, Alkaline, and Watery Recipes to Prevent Heartburn and Nourish Your Gut-Includes a 60-Day Meal Plan for All Stages

ETHEL LEMKE

TABLE OF CONTENTS

INTRODUCTION

Imagine a life where vibrant meals don't trigger your acid reflux, but soothe it. As a doctor and registered dietitian who's spent over a decade helping people just like you, I know how frustrating and limiting GERD can feel. I've seen firsthand how the endless cycle of bland, restrictive diets and the constant fear of flare-ups can take a toll on your joy of eating.

But let me tell you something from the heart: it doesn't have to be this way. My years of experience have taught me that food can be both a source of immense pleasure and a powerful healer. I've spent countless hours in the kitchen, experimenting with recipes and researching the science behind GERD triggers, and I've discovered that delicious meals and a happy gut can go hand-in-hand.

This cookbook isn't just another collection of recipes. It's a testament to the fact that you can reclaim your love of food without sacrificing your health. It's a culinary roadmap that will lead you through a flavorful adventure, where we'll explore the science behind GERD, uncover the power of nutrient-dense ingredients, and unlock the joy of preparing meals that taste as good as they make you feel.

I'm not promising you a miracle cure, but I am promising you this: this cookbook will empower you to make informed choices, discover new flavors, and rediscover the simple pleasure of eating without fear. Together, we'll transform your relationship with food, one delicious bite at a time. So, get ready to say goodbye to bland diets and hello to a life where every meal is a celebration of flavor, health, and the joy of eating.

CHAPTER 1

DECODING ACID REFLUX AND GERD: THE INSIDE SCOOP

Ever had that fiery feeling in your chest after a delicious meal? Or perhaps that sour taste creeping up your throat when you're trying to sleep? Chances are, you've experienced acid reflux – a common but uncomfortable condition where stomach acid backflows into your esophagus (the tube connecting your mouth to your stomach). Think of it like a wave washing back up the beach instead of receding; it's not supposed to happen, and it can leave a bit of a sting.

Let's break it down. Your stomach is a powerful organ that churns and digests food with the help of acid. Usually, a tight muscle called the lower esophageal sphincter (LES) acts like a one-way door, keeping the acid where it belongs – in your stomach. But sometimes, this door gets a bit lazy or weak, allowing acid to sneak back up into the esophagus, leading to that burning sensation we all know as heartburn.

GERD, or gastroesophageal reflux disease, is essentially acid reflux on repeat. Instead of just an occasional annoyance, it's a chronic issue where the backflow of acid happens frequently, causing not only heartburn but also potentially damaging the delicate lining of your esophagus. Think of it like a persistent drizzle versus a sudden downpour; the drizzle might be manageable, but over time, it can erode the landscape.

So, how can you tell if you're dealing with occasional reflux or full-blown GERD?

- **Occasional Reflux:** You might feel heartburn sporadically, usually triggered by specific foods, large meals, or lying down too soon after eating. It's a nuisance, but not a daily struggle.
- **GERD:** If heartburn strikes more than twice a week, wakes you up at night, or comes with other symptoms like regurgitation (that sour taste in your mouth), chest pain, or difficulty swallowing, it's time to pay closer attention. Your body is trying to tell you something.

Why Does This Happen?

There are a few usual suspects:

1. **A Weak LES:** Sometimes, that muscular door at the bottom of your esophagus simply doesn't close as tightly as it should, allowing acid to escape.
2. **Hiatal Hernia:** This happens when the upper part of your stomach pushes through a weak spot in your diaphragm (the muscle that separates your chest from your abdomen). This can put pressure on the LES and make it harder to do its job.
3. **Lifestyle Factors:** Certain habits like smoking, excessive alcohol consumption, and late-night eating can all weaken the LES and trigger reflux.
4. **Pregnancy and Weight Gain:** Changes in your body, like weight gain or pregnancy, can increase pressure on your stomach and make it easier for acid to back up.

Don't Worry, You're Not Alone

The good news is that you're not alone in this. Millions of people experience acid reflux and GERD. And while there's no one-size-fits-all solution, there are many effective ways to manage symptoms and improve your quality of life.

In the next chapter, we'll dive deeper into the warning signs of GERD and explore how you can take control of your health through dietary changes, lifestyle adjustments, and, if needed, medication. Remember, knowledge is power. By understanding what's happening in your body, you can make informed choices that will lead to a happier, healthier you.

Your Food's Journey:

Alright, let's get real about how your gut works. When you eat, your food travels down your esophagus, a tube that connects your mouth to your stomach. Your stomach is like a powerful blender, using strong acids to break down food.

Now, there's a little muscle at the bottom of your esophagus called the lower esophageal sphincter (LES). Think of it as a one-way door that's supposed to let food into your stomach and then close tightly to keep the acid inside.

But sometimes, that door doesn't do its job very well. It can get weak or loose, letting stomach acid sneak back up into your esophagus. That's what causes that burning sensation we call heartburn.

When this happens a lot – more than a couple of times a week – it's called GERD (gastroesophageal reflux disease). It's like having a leaky faucet; it's not just a one-time spill, but a constant drip that can cause real problems over time.

So, what makes that door get lazy? A few things can contribute:

- **Hiatal Hernia:** This is when the upper part of your stomach pushes up through your diaphragm (the muscle that separates your chest from your belly). It's like having a bulge in a garden hose; it can mess with the flow and make it harder for the door to close properly.
- **Extra Weight or Pregnancy:** Carrying extra pounds or having a growing baby can put pressure on your stomach, making it easier for acid to escape.
- **Lifestyle Habits:** Smoking, drinking too much alcohol, and late-night eating can all weaken that door, like leaving it unlocked and inviting trouble inside.

Now, here's the thing: GERD isn't just about heartburn. It can also cause other annoying symptoms like:

- **A Scratchy, Irritated Throat:** That acid can travel all the way up to your throat, causing a persistent cough or a feeling that something's stuck.
- **Trouble Breathing:** In some cases, the acid can even reach your lungs, triggering wheezing and shortness of breath.
- **Sour or Bitter Taste:** If you wake up with a nasty taste in your mouth, it could be acid that crept up while you were sleeping.

If you're experiencing any of these symptoms, don't brush them off. Talk to your doctor to get a proper diagnosis and discuss the best ways to manage your GERD.

Remember, you're not alone in this. Millions of people deal with GERD, and there are plenty of effective solutions. In the next chapters, we'll explore foods that can soothe your symptoms, lifestyle changes that can make a big difference, and medications that can help if needed. You've got this!

CHAPTER 2

EATING FOR A HAPPY GUT: YOUR GERD-FRIENDLY GUIDE

Let's be honest, food is meant to be enjoyed. But when you're dealing with GERD, some of our favorite treats can feel like they're throwing a party in your esophagus...and not the fun kind. It's like adding fuel to an already burning fire. The good news is that by understanding which foods tend to be troublemakers, you can make choices that actually help you feel better, not worse.

The Fatty Food Fiasco

First up on the list are fatty foods. Think of your lower esophageal sphincter (LES) – that little door between your esophagus and stomach – as a muscle. Fatty foods tend to make that muscle relax and get a bit lazy, making it easier for stomach acid to sneak back up. Plus, they slow down digestion, meaning food hangs out in your stomach longer, increasing the pressure and making backflow more likely.

Here are some of the usual suspects:

- **Fast Food Favorites:** Fried chicken, French fries, greasy burgers – these are loaded with the kind of fats that can trigger heartburn.
- **Snack Attackers:** Potato chips, processed snacks, and ice cream might be tempting, but they're also packed with fats that can wreak havoc on your gut.
- **Rich and Creamy Delights:** Full-fat dairy products like whole milk, cheese, and sour cream can increase stomach acid and weaken your LES.
- **Fatty Cuts of Meat:** Bacon, sausage, and marbled steaks might be delicious, but their high fat content makes them a risky choice for those with GERD.

- **The Egg Enigma:** Egg whites are generally safe, but those rich, yellow yolks are high in fat. This can slow down digestion and make reflux more likely. Fried eggs are a double whammy, adding even more fat to the mix.

The Spice Situation

Spicy foods are a bit of a mixed bag. They don't directly cause acid reflux, but they can irritate an already inflamed esophagus. It's like pouring lemon juice on a paper cut; it might not cause the cut, but it sure doesn't help it heal!

Here are some spices to approach with caution:

- **Chili Powders:** Cayenne pepper, black pepper, white pepper – they add heat, but they can also turn up the heat on your existing reflux symptoms.
- **Curry Dishes:** Even if a curry isn't super spicy, some of the spice blends can be irritating to a sensitive esophagus.

I know it can feel overwhelming to think about cutting back on some of your favorite foods. But remember, this isn't about deprivation, it's about making smart choices that will help you feel your best. And the good news is, there are plenty of delicious and satisfying options that are gentle on your gut. We'll explore those in the next chapter, so stay tuned!

The Acidic Culprits: Fruits, Veggies, & Beverages

Now, here's where it gets a bit tricky. Fruits and vegetables are super important for good health, but some can be sneaky troublemakers when it comes to acid reflux. It's like having a friend who means well but always seems to spill their drink on you at parties.

Citrus Powerhouses: Oranges, grapefruits, lemons, and limes are packed with vitamin C, but their high acidity can irritate your esophagus and relax that little trapdoor (LES) we talked about.

Tomato Trap: As much as we love them on pizza and in pasta sauce, tomatoes – even cooked ones – can be a major trigger for many people with GERD.

Sneaky Onions & Garlic: These guys add flavor to so many dishes, but they can also worsen symptoms for some folks, especially when eaten raw.

Beverage Battle: Bubbly drinks like soda and sparkling water can create pressure in your stomach, making acid reflux more likely. Alcohol, coffee (even decaf!), and citrus juices are also common culprits.

Everyone's Different: Remember, not everyone reacts the same way to these foods. Some people can tolerate them just fine, while others need to avoid them altogether. It's all about paying attention to how your body reacts and finding what works for you.

Portion Sizes Matter: Even "safe" foods can become a problem if you eat too much at once. It's like filling a bathtub to the brim – eventually, it's going to overflow. So, try to enjoy these foods in moderation.

Foods That Fight Back: Soothing & Alkaline-Forming Heroes

But don't worry, it's not all doom and gloom! There are plenty of delicious and satisfying foods that can actually help soothe your symptoms and keep your gut happy.

Fiber-tastic Foods: Think of fiber as a sponge that helps absorb stomach acid and keep things moving smoothly through your digestive system. Good sources include:

- **Fruits & Vegetables:** Leafy greens, melons, and most other non-citrus fruits and veggies are packed with fiber and nutrients.
- **Whole Grains:** Whole-wheat bread, brown rice, quinoa, and oats will keep you feeling full and satisfied, reducing the urge to overeat (which can trigger reflux).

- **Beans & Legumes:** Lentils, chickpeas, and black beans are fiber powerhouses that also offer a good dose of protein.

Alkaline Allies: These foods help neutralize excess acid in your stomach and esophagus:

- **Melons:** Watermelon, honeydew, and cantaloupe are not only refreshing but also naturally low in acid.
- **Bananas:** Ripe bananas are easy on the stomach and have an alkalizing effect.
- **Leafy Greens:** Spinach, kale, and other leafy greens are packed with alkaline minerals that can help balance your pH levels.

The Soothing Stars: These foods help coat and protect your esophagus, reducing irritation:

- **Oatmeal:** This comforting classic is like a warm hug for your tummy. It absorbs acid and promotes healthy digestion.
- **Ginger:** Ginger has natural anti-inflammatory properties that can help calm an upset stomach and reduce nausea.
- **Avocados:** These creamy fruits are packed with healthy fats that are easy to digest and won't trigger reflux.

Watery Wonders: Staying hydrated is crucial for good digestion and can help dilute stomach acid. Good options include:

- **Herbal Teas:** Chamomile and ginger teas are soothing and caffeine-free.
- **Plant-Based Milks:** Unsweetened almond milk, coconut milk, and oat milk are great alternatives to dairy if you're sensitive to it.
- **Non-Acidic Juices:** Carrot juice and other vegetable juices can provide nutrients without the acidic bite of citrus fruits.

Your GERD-Friendly Food List: Building a Happy Gut Pantry

This chart is your guide to choosing foods that are not only delicious but also gentle on your stomach and esophagus. Remember, everyone's body is different, so it's important to listen to your own and see how you react to different foods.

Food Category	Examples	Why They're Good for GERD	Tips and Considerations
Soothing & Alkaline	Melons (all kinds), bananas, leafy greens	Help neutralize stomach acid, reduce inflammation, and soothe the esophagus	Enjoy them raw, cooked, or blended into smoothies.
Watery Wonders	Herbal teas (chamomile, ginger), plant-based milks (unsweetened), non-acidic juices (carrot, veggie)	Help dilute stomach acid and keep you hydrated without triggering reflux	Choose unsweetened varieties and limit fruit juices to small amounts.
Fiber Powerhouses	Whole grains (oats, brown rice, quinoa), beans & legumes (lentils, chickpeas), broccoli, cauliflower, asparagus, beans, potatoes (with skin), cucumbers, berries, pears, apples	Fiber helps absorb stomach acid and keeps things moving smoothly through your digestive system.	Aim for a variety of fiber sources throughout the day.

Protein Picks	Lean chicken & turkey, fish & seafood, egg whites, tofu & tempeh	Provide essential nutrients without the high fat content that can trigger reflux	Grill, bake, or poach for healthier cooking methods.
Healthy Fats	Avocados, walnuts, flaxseeds, olive oil, sesame oil, sunflower oil	Promote satiety and help absorb fat-soluble vitamins without aggravating GERD	Use in moderation as part of a balanced meal.

Important Note: This is just a starting point! There are many other delicious and GERD-friendly foods out there. Don't be afraid to experiment and discover new favorites.

CHAPTER 3

BEYOND THE PLATE: LIFESTYLE CHANGES TO CONQUER GERD

Eating right is a major step towards managing GERD, but it's not the only one. The way you live your life plays a huge role in how you feel, especially when it comes to acid reflux. It's time to look beyond your plate and explore some lifestyle changes that can make a real difference.

Stress: The Silent Saboteur

Stress isn't just a mental thing; it can wreak havoc on your whole body, including your gut. When you're stressed, your body goes into fight-or-flight mode, pumping out hormones that can tighten your muscles (including your LES!), increase stomach acid production, and make you more sensitive to GERD symptoms. It's like adding lighter fluid to an already smoldering fire.

But don't worry, there are ways to fight back:

- **Move Your Body:** Gentle exercise like walking, yoga, or stretching can help relax both your mind and body, reducing stress hormones and easing tension.
- **Breathe Deep:** Taking slow, deep breaths activates your parasympathetic nervous system, which is like your body's built-in "chill-out" button.
- **Make Time for Relaxation:** Find activities that help you unwind and de-stress, whether it's reading a book, taking a bath, or listening to calming music. Make them a regular part of your routine.

Sleep: Your Gut's Best Friend

Sleep and GERD have a complicated relationship. Reflux can keep you up at night, and poor sleep can make your GERD worse. Here's how to create a better sleep environment for your gut:

- **Position is Key:** Lying flat makes it easier for stomach acid to creep up into your esophagus. Elevate the head of your bed by about 6-8 inches with blocks or a wedge pillow.
- **Sleep on Your Left Side:** This position can help keep your stomach below your esophagus, reducing the chance of acid backflow.
- **Timing Matters:** Avoid eating large meals or spicy foods within 3 hours of bedtime. Give your stomach a chance to empty before you lie down.
- **Prioritize Sleep Quality:** Aim for 7-8 hours of good sleep every night. Being well-rested allows your body to repair and function optimally, including managing GERD symptoms.

Weight Management: Take the Pressure Off

Carrying extra weight, especially around your midsection, puts pressure on your stomach, making it easier for acid to escape. Even losing a small amount of weight can make a significant difference in your symptoms.

- **Focus on Sustainable Changes:** Crash diets can stress your body and often lead to rebound weight gain. Instead, make gradual changes to your eating habits and activity levels that you can stick with long-term.
- **Move More, Choose Wisely:** Increase your physical activity and focus on whole, unprocessed foods. These small changes can add up to big results over time.
- **Get Support:** If you need help developing a weight loss plan that's safe and effective for GERD, talk to a registered dietitian.

Habits to Kick: Ditch the GERD Triggers

Certain habits can be the best friends of acid reflux. It's time to say goodbye to these troublemakers:

- **Smoking:** This is a major no-no for anyone with GERD. Smoking weakens your LES, damages your esophagus, and increases your risk of complications. Quitting is the single best thing you can do for your gut health (and your overall health!).
- **Alcohol:** Alcohol relaxes your LES, irritates your stomach lining, and can disrupt your sleep – a recipe for reflux disaster. Limit your intake or avoid it altogether, especially close to bedtime.
- **Late-Night Eating:** Eating a big meal right before bed is like setting the stage for heartburn. Give your stomach at least 3 hours to digest before lying down.

The Bottom Line:

Managing GERD isn't just about what you eat. It's about how you live. By prioritizing stress management, good sleep, a healthy weight, and ditching those bad habits, you can significantly reduce your symptoms and improve your overall quality of life.

Remember, every small change counts. You don't have to do it all at once. Start with one or two changes and gradually incorporate more as you go. Your gut will thank you!

CHAPTER 4

THE RECIPE COLLECTION

BREAKFASTS

BANANA BERRY BLAST SMOOTHIE

Prep time: 5 minutes | **Serving size:** 1 | **Special considerations:** Gluten-free, vegetarian, vegan, budget-friendly

Why It's a GERD-Friendly Winner

Bananas and berries are your gut's best friends! They're naturally low in acid, high in fiber (hello, smooth digestion!), and bursting with antioxidants that fight inflammation.

INGREDIENTS

- 1 frozen banana, sliced
- 1 cup packed spinach or kale (fresh or frozen)
- 1 cup mixed berries (blueberries, raspberries, strawberries – whatever you have on hand!)
- 1 cup unsweetened almond milk (or your favorite non-dairy milk)
- ½ teaspoon ground cinnamon (optional, for a warming touch)

INSTRUCTIONS

1. Toss everything into a blender.
2. Blend until smooth and creamy. If it's too thick, add a splash more milk.
3. Pour into a glass and enjoy!

- Frozen fruit is key for a thick, frosty smoothie. No frozen bananas? Use a fresh one and toss in a few ice cubes.
- Don't have kale? Spinach works just as well.
- Want to make it even more filling? Add a scoop of protein powder or a tablespoon of nut butter.

APPROXIMATE NUTRITIONAL INFO (PER SERVING)

Calories: 250

Protein: 8g

Fiber: 10g

Healthy Fats: 5g

Potassium: 600mg

TROPICAL GREEN DREAM SMOOTHIE

Prep time: 5 minutes | **Serving size**: 1 | **Special considerations:** Gluten-free, vegetarian, vegan

Why It's a GERD-Friendly Winner

This smoothie is like a vacation for your gut! Mango and avocado are alkaline-forming (meaning they help neutralize stomach acid), while avocado's healthy fats keep you feeling full without triggering reflux. Plus, turmeric adds a powerful anti-inflammatory punch.

INGREDIENTS

- 1 cup frozen mango chunks
- ½ avocado, peeled and pitted
- 1 cup packed spinach (fresh or frozen)
- ½ cup non-dairy yogurt (coconut or almond)
- 1 cup unsweetened coconut milk
- ¼ teaspoon ground turmeric

INSTRUCTIONS

1. Combine all ingredients in a blender.
2. Blend until smooth and creamy.
3. Pour into a glass and enjoy this tropical escape!

- Adjust the sweetness to your liking with a drizzle of honey or maple syrup.
- Sprinkle with unsweetened coconut flakes or a few chunks of fresh pineapple for a truly tropical experience.
- Add a handful of kale or other leafy greens for an extra nutrient boost.

APPROXIMATE NUTRITIONAL INFO (PER SERVING)

- Calories: 350
- Protein: 7g
- Fiber: 12g
- Healthy Fats: 20g
- Vitamin C: 80% Daily Value

CREAMY GINGER PEACH SMOOTHIE

Prep time: 10 minutes (includes soaking time for oats) | **Serving size**: 1 | **Special considerations:** Gluten-free, vegetarian, vegan

Why It's a GERD-Friendly Winner

This smoothie is a powerhouse of soothing ingredients. Ginger helps reduce inflammation and aids digestion, while rolled oats provide gentle fiber and absorb excess stomach acid. Peaches offer natural sweetness without the acidity of citrus fruits.

INGREDIENTS

- 1 cup frozen peaches, sliced
- ½ avocado, peeled and pitted
- 1 tablespoon grated fresh ginger
- ½ cup non-dairy milk (almond, oat, etc.)
- ¼ cup rolled oats
- ½ teaspoon ground cinnamon
- Optional: 1-2 Medjool dates for extra sweetness

INSTRUCTIONS

1. Soak rolled oats in water for 10-15 minutes. This will make them easier to digest.
2. Drain the oats and combine all ingredients in a blender.
3. Blend until smooth and creamy.
4. Enjoy the creamy, soothing goodness!

TIPS

- Use fresh peaches when they're in season or frozen peaches year-round.
- Add a pinch of cardamom or nutmeg for extra warmth and spice.
- Swap non-dairy milk for a dollop of non-dairy yogurt for a richer texture.

APPROXIMATE NUTRITIONAL INFO (PER SERVING)

- Calories: 300 (without dates)
- Protein: 6g
- Fiber: 10g
- Healthy Fats: 15g
- Vitamin A: 30% Daily Value

BLUEBERRY BLISS OATMEAL

Prep time: 5 minutes | **Cook time:** 5-7 minutes | **Serving size:** 1 | **Special considerations:**
Gluten-free (if using certified gluten-free oats), vegetarian, vegan | **Budget-friendly tip:**
Purchase rolled oats in bulk for a more economical option

Why It's a GERD-Friendly Winner

Rolled oats are a gentle hug for your stomach, providing soothing fiber that helps absorb excess acid and keeps you feeling full. Blueberries bring a burst of sweetness and antioxidants without the acidic punch of citrus fruits. A sprinkle of almonds adds healthy fats and a satisfying crunch.

INGREDIENTS

- ½ cup rolled oats
- 1 cup unsweetened almond milk (or your preferred milk)
- ¼ cup blueberries (fresh or frozen)
- 1 tablespoon chia seeds
- ½ teaspoon maple syrup (optional)
- 1 tablespoon sliced almonds

INSTRUCTIONS

1. In a small saucepan, combine oats, almond milk, blueberries, and chia seeds.
2. Bring to a simmer over medium heat, then reduce heat to low and cook for 5-7 minutes, stirring occasionally, until oatmeal is thickened and creamy.
3. Remove from heat and stir in maple syrup if desired.
4. Top with sliced almonds and enjoy warm.

- Get creative with toppings: Swap almonds for walnuts or pecans, add a sprinkle of pumpkin seeds, or a drizzle of honey.
- Add a fruity twist: Stir in a spoonful of mashed banana or diced apple for extra flavor and sweetness.
- Make-ahead option: Prepare overnight oats by combining all ingredients (except toppings) in a jar and refrigerating overnight. Enjoy cold or gently reheat in the morning.

APPROXIMATE NUTRITIONAL INFO (PER SERVING)

- Calories: 320
- Protein: 10g
- Fiber: 12g
- Healthy Fats: 12g
- Iron: 15% Daily Value

APPLE SPICE DELIGHT OATMEAL

Prep time: 5 minutes | **Cook time:** 5-7 minutes | **Serving size:** 1 | **Special considerations:** Gluten-free (if using certified gluten-free oats), vegetarian, vegan | **Budget-friendly tip:** Use in-season apples for the best flavor and value

Why It's a GERD-Friendly Winner

This warm and comforting oatmeal is perfect for cooler mornings. Apples add natural sweetness and fiber without the acidity of citrus fruits. The cinnamon and nutmeg create a cozy flavor profile that won't irritate your esophagus.

INGREDIENTS

- ½ cup rolled oats
- 1 cup unsweetened vanilla almond milk (or your preferred milk)
- ½ apple, peeled and finely grated
- ½ teaspoon ground cinnamon
- Pinch of ground nutmeg
- 1 tablespoon chopped walnuts

INSTRUCTIONS

1. In a small saucepan, combine oats, almond milk, grated apple, cinnamon, and nutmeg.
2. Bring to a simmer over medium heat, then reduce heat to low and cook for 5-7 minutes, stirring frequently, until oatmeal thickens and the apple is tender.
3. Pour into a bowl and top with chopped walnuts.

TIPS

- Choose your apple wisely: Opt for a sweeter variety like Gala or Honeycrisp for extra flavor.
- Play with texture: Grate the apple coarsely for more texture, or use applesauce if you prefer a smoother consistency.
- Experiment with flavors: Add a pinch of ginger for warmth or a swirl of your favorite nut butter for extra richness.

APPROXIMATE NUTRITIONAL INFO (PER SERVING)

- Calories: 300
- Protein: 8g
- Fiber: 10g
- Healthy Fats: 10g
- Manganese: 50% Daily Value

SAVORY SUNSHINE BOWL

Prep time: 5 minutes | **Cook time:** 10 minutes | **Serving size:** 1 | **Special considerations:** Gluten-free (if using certified gluten-free oats), vegetarian | Budget-friendly tip: If you have leftover cooked quinoa or brown rice, you can substitute it for the oats

Why It's a GERD-Friendly Winner

This savory twist on oatmeal is packed with protein and veggies. Zucchini and turmeric offer antioxidants and anti-inflammatory benefits, while the egg white provides lean protein to keep you feeling full and energized.

INGREDIENTS

- ½ cup rolled oats
- 1 cup vegetable broth
- ¼ cup grated zucchini
- ¼ teaspoon ground turmeric
- Pinch of black pepper
- 1 egg white
- Optional toppings: sliced avocado, chopped fresh herbs (cilantro, parsley)

INSTRUCTIONS

1. In a small saucepan, combine oats and vegetable broth.
2. Bring to a simmer over medium heat, then reduce heat to low, stir in grated zucchini and turmeric, and cook for 5-7 minutes, or until the oats are tender and most of the liquid is absorbed.
3. Season with black pepper.
4. While the oats are cooking, poach the egg white.
5. Top the oatmeal with the poached egg white and any desired toppings.

- Change up the veggies: Swap zucchini for broccoli florets, chopped spinach, or other GERD-friendly vegetables.
- Add a burst of freshness: Top with your favorite chopped fresh herbs like cilantro, parsley, or chives.
- Spice it up (if tolerated): A pinch of red pepper flakes can add a subtle kick if you can handle a little spice.

APPROXIMATE NUTRITIONAL INFO (PER SERVING)

- Calories: 250
- Protein: 15g
- Fiber: 8g
- Healthy Fats: 8g
- Iron: 20% Daily Value

SPINACH & FETA SCRAMBLE

Prep time: 5 minutes | **Cook time:** 5 minutes | **Serving size:** 1 | **Special considerations:** Gluten-free, high in protein, low in fat, vegetarian | **Budget-friendly tip:** Feta can be pricey. Swap it for a sprinkle of parmesan cheese or a dollop of cottage cheese for a similar flavor profile.

Why It's a GERD-Friendly Winner

This simple scramble is packed with protein from egg whites, fiber from spinach, and a touch of savory flavor from feta cheese. It's a light and satisfying way to start your day without triggering reflux.

INGREDIENTS

- 4 large egg whites
- ½ cup chopped spinach (fresh or frozen)
- 1 tablespoon crumbled feta cheese
- 1 teaspoon chopped fresh dill (or ½ teaspoon dried dill)
- Salt and pepper to taste
- 1 slice whole-grain toast

INSTRUCTIONS

1. In a bowl, whisk together egg whites, spinach, feta, dill, salt, and pepper.
2. Heat a small non-stick skillet over medium heat.
3. Pour in the egg mixture and cook, gently stirring, until the eggs are set and cooked through (about 3-5 minutes).
4. Serve immediately with a slice of toasted whole-grain bread.

TIPS

- Veggie Variety: Swap spinach for chopped zucchini, bell peppers, or mushrooms.

- Add a Kick: If you tolerate spice, add a pinch of red pepper flakes for a little heat.

- Make-Ahead Option: Prepare the scramble in advance and reheat gently in the microwave.

APPROXIMATE NUTRITIONAL INFO (PER SERVING)

- Calories: 200
- Protein: 20g
- Fiber: 4g
- Healthy Fats: 5g
- Calcium: 15% Daily Value

VEGGIE-PACKED FRITTATA BITES

Prep time: 10 minutes | **Cook time:** 15-20 minutes | **Serving size:** 6 frittata bites (2-3 bites per serving) | **Special considerations:** Gluten-free, dairy-free (if omitting cheese), high in protein, vegetarian | **Budget-friendly tip:** Use seasonal vegetables or whatever you have on hand to keep costs down

Why It's a GERD-Friendly Winner

These mini frittatas are like a flavor explosion in every bite! Packed with veggies and protein from egg whites, they're a delicious and convenient way to start your day on the right foot.

INGREDIENTS

- 6 large egg whites
- ½ cup chopped broccoli florets
- ¼ cup chopped bell pepper (any color)
- ¼ cup chopped onion
- Salt and pepper to taste
- Optional: A sprinkle of feta cheese or a pinch of grated parmesan

INSTRUCTIONS

1. Preheat oven to 350°F (175°C). Grease a muffin tin.
2. In a bowl, whisk together egg whites, broccoli, bell pepper, onion, salt, and pepper.
3. Divide the mixture evenly among the muffin cups. Sprinkle with cheese if desired.
4. Bake for 15-20 minutes, or until the eggs are set and slightly puffed.
5. Let cool slightly before removing from the muffin tin.

- Endless Veggie Options: Get creative with your fillings! Try mushrooms, spinach, zucchini, or even leftover cooked sweet potato.
- Meal Prep Power: These frittatas keep well in the refrigerator for a few days and are perfect for on-the-go breakfasts or snacks.
- Herb It Up: A sprinkle of fresh herbs like parsley, dill, or chives adds a burst of flavor.

APPROXIMATE NUTRITIONAL INFO (PER SERVING)

- Calories: 100
- Protein: 10g
- Fiber: 3g
- Healthy Fats: 2g
- Vitamin C: 40% Daily Value

BANANA BUCKWHEAT PANCAKES

Prep time: 10 minutes | **Cook time:** 10 minutes | **Serving size:** 2-3 pancakes | **Special considerations:** Gluten-free, vegetarian, vegan-adaptable (use a flaxseed "egg" instead of egg whites) | **Budget-friendly tip:** Buckwheat flour can be found in bulk bins at many grocery stores, saving you money compared to pre-packaged options

Why It's a GERD-Friendly Winner

These fluffy pancakes are made with buckwheat flour, a naturally gluten-free grain that's high in fiber and gentle on the stomach. The sweetness comes from mashed bananas, avoiding the acidic punch of refined sugars. Egg whites provide protein without the fat found in yolks.

INGREDIENTS

- ½ cup buckwheat flour
- 1 ripe banana, mashed
- 2 egg whites (or 1 flaxseed "egg" for vegan option)
- ½ cup unsweetened almond milk (or your preferred milk)
- ¼ teaspoon baking soda
- ¼ teaspoon ground cinnamon
- Optional: Maple syrup, honey, or berries for serving

INSTRUCTIONS

1. In a bowl, whisk together buckwheat flour, mashed banana, egg whites (or flaxseed "egg"), almond milk, baking soda, and cinnamon until well combined.
2. Heat a lightly oiled griddle or non-stick skillet over medium heat.
3. Pour ¼ cup portions of batter onto the griddle for each pancake.
4. Cook for 2-3 minutes per side, or until golden brown and cooked through.
5. Serve warm with your favorite toppings.

TIPS

- If you're using a flaxseed "egg," combine 1 tablespoon ground flaxseed with 3 tablespoons water and let sit for 5 minutes before using.
- For extra flavor and texture, fold a few blueberries or chopped nuts into the batter before cooking.
- Leftover pancakes can be stored in the refrigerator or freezer for a quick and easy breakfast.

APPROXIMATE NUTRITIONAL INFO (PER SERVING)

- Calories: 200
- Protein: 8g
- Fiber: 6g
- Healthy Fats: 4g
- Manganese: 50% Daily Value

SWEET POTATO HASH WITH TURKEY SAUSAGE AND SAGE

Prep time: 10 minutes (plus any pre-cooking time for the sweet potatoes) | **Cook time:** 10-15 minutes | **Serving size:** 2 | **Special considerations:** Gluten-free, dairy-free, paleo-friendly | **Budget-friendly tip:** Buy sweet potatoes in bulk and roast a large batch for the week. They'll last in the refrigerator for several days and can be used in various dishes

Why It's a GERD-Friendly Winner

This savory breakfast hash is packed with fiber-rich sweet potatoes, lean protein from turkey sausage, and the anti-inflammatory benefits of sage. It's a satisfying and flavorful way to fuel your morning.

INGREDIENTS

- 1 ½ cups cooked and cubed sweet potato (boiled or roasted)
- ½ cup cooked lean turkey sausage, crumbled
- ½ cup chopped green beans
- ½ teaspoon dried sage
- Salt and pepper to taste
- Optional: 1 tablespoon olive oil for cooking

INSTRUCTIONS

1. Heat a large skillet over medium heat. Add olive oil if desired.
2. Add the sweet potato cubes and turkey sausage and cook until heated through, about 5 minutes.
3. Stir in the green beans and sage and cook for another 5-7 minutes, or until the beans are tender-crisp.
4. Season with salt and pepper to taste.

- For a vegetarian option, substitute the turkey sausage with plant-based sausage or crumbled tofu.
- Feel free to add other GERD-friendly vegetables like chopped kale, spinach, or mushrooms.
- Experiment with different herbs and spices to customize the flavor.

APPROXIMATE NUTRITIONAL INFO (PER SERVING)

- Calories: 250
- Protein: 20g
- Fiber: 6g
- Healthy Fats: 5g
- Vitamin A: 150% Daily Value

AVOCADO TOAST DELUXE

Prep time: 5 minutes | **Cook time:** 5 minutes (for poaching the egg) | **Serving size:** 1 | **Special considerations:** Gluten-free (if using gluten-free bread), vegetarian | **Budget-friendly tip:** Buy avocados when they're in season for the best price and flavor

Why It's a GERD-Friendly Winner

This elevated avocado toast is a delicious and nutritious way to start your day. Avocado provides healthy fats and fiber, while the whole-grain toast offers complex carbohydrates for sustained energy. The poached egg white adds a boost of lean protein.

INGREDIENTS

- 1 slice whole-grain bread, toasted
- ¼ avocado, mashed
- 1 poached egg white
- Pinch of salt, black pepper, and red pepper flakes (optional)
- 1 tablespoon hemp seeds

INSTRUCTIONS

1. Toast the bread.
2. While the bread is toasting, poach the egg white.
3. Spread the mashed avocado evenly over the toast.
4. Top with the poached egg white.
5. Season with salt, pepper, and red pepper flakes (if using).
6. Sprinkle with hemp seeds.

- Experiment with different types of whole-grain bread, such as sourdough, rye, or multigrain.
- Add a squeeze of lemon juice, a drizzle of balsamic glaze, or a sprinkle of your favorite herbs for extra flavor.
- If you're not comfortable poaching an egg, you can try scrambling the egg white or cooking it sunny-side up.

APPROXIMATE NUTRITIONAL INFO (PER SERVING)

- Calories: 300
- Protein: 15g
- Fiber: 8g
- Healthy Fats: 15g
- Vitamin E: 30% Daily Value

MELON & MINT SALAD

Prep time: 5 minutes | **Serving size:** 1 | **Special considerations:** Vegan, gluten-free, low in calories, naturally sweet | **Budget-friendly tip:** Choose melons that are in season for the best flavor and price

Why It's a GERD-Friendly Winner

This refreshing and hydrating salad is a perfect way to start your day. Melons like watermelon, cantaloupe, and honeydew are naturally alkaline and low in acid, making them gentle on your stomach. Mint adds a cool, invigorating flavor and can help soothe digestion.

INGREDIENTS

- 1 cup cubed watermelon
- 1 cup cubed honeydew or cantaloupe
- ¼ cup fresh mint leaves, chopped
- 1 tablespoon plain non-dairy yogurt (optional)

INSTRUCTIONS

1. Combine cubed watermelon, honeydew (or cantaloupe), and chopped mint in a bowl.
2. If desired, top with a dollop of non-dairy yogurt.

TIPS

- Mix it up: Use any combination of your favorite melons for a colorful and flavorful salad.
- Add a touch of sweetness: If you prefer a sweeter salad, drizzle a small amount of honey or maple syrup on top.
- Experiment with yogurt: Try different flavors of non-dairy yogurt like vanilla or coconut for variety.

APPROXIMATE NUTRITIONAL INFO (PER SERVING)

- Calories: 100
- Protein: 2g
- Fiber: 3g
- Healthy Fats: 0g
- Vitamin C: 50% Daily Value

CUCUMBER & CHIA DELIGHT

Prep time: 5 minutes (plus overnight soaking time) | **Serving size:** 1 | **Special considerations:** Vegan, gluten-free, high in fiber | **Budget-friendly tip:** Chia seeds are a cost-effective source of fiber and omega-3 fatty acids.

Why It's a GERD-Friendly Winner

This simple yet satisfying breakfast is packed with nutrients and gentle on your stomach. Chia seeds are loaded with fiber and healthy fats, while cucumber is hydrating and soothing for digestion. The banana adds natural sweetness, and the almond milk provides a creamy base.

INGREDIENTS

- 2 tablespoons chia seeds
- 1 cup unsweetened almond milk (or your preferred milk)
- ½ cup chopped cucumber
- ½ ripe banana, sliced
- 1 teaspoon honey (optional)

INSTRUCTIONS

1. The night before, combine chia seeds and almond milk in a jar or container. Stir well.
2. Refrigerate overnight (or for at least 30 minutes). The chia seeds will absorb the liquid and create a pudding-like consistency.
3. In the morning, stir the chia pudding mixture.
4. Layer with chopped cucumber, sliced banana, and a drizzle of honey if desired.

- Prep for the week: Make a larger batch of chia pudding to enjoy throughout the week.
- Vary your toppings: Try different fruits like berries or mango, or add a sprinkle of granola for extra crunch.
- Flavor it up: Stir in a pinch of cinnamon, a dash of vanilla extract, or a few drops of almond extract for extra flavor.

APPROXIMATE NUTRITIONAL INFO (PER SERVING)

- Calories: 250
- Protein: 7g
- Fiber: 12g
- Healthy Fats: 10g
- Calcium: 30% Daily Value

SIMPLE GREEN GOODNESS

Prep time: 5 minutes | **Serving size:** 1 | **Special considerations:** Vegan, gluten-free, low in calories | **Budget-friendly tip:** Buy leafy greens in bulk or grow your own to save money

Why It's a GERD-Friendly Winner

This light and refreshing salad is packed with nutrients and easy to digest. Leafy greens are a great source of fiber and alkaline minerals, while avocado and olive oil provide healthy fats. The lemon juice adds a bright, zesty flavor, and sunflower seeds provide a satisfying crunch.

INGREDIENTS

- 2 cups mixed leafy greens (spinach, kale, arugula, etc.)
- 1 tablespoon olive oil
- 1 squeeze lemon juice
- ¼ cup sunflower seeds
- 2 slices cooked turkey bacon, crumbled (optional)

INSTRUCTIONS

1. In a bowl, combine leafy greens, olive oil, and lemon juice. Toss to coat.
2. Top with sunflower seeds and crumbled turkey bacon (if using).

TIPS

- Mix and match greens: Use any combination of your favorite leafy greens for a variety of flavors and textures.
- Get creative with toppings: Swap sunflower seeds for pumpkin seeds, chopped walnuts, or a sprinkle of hemp seeds.
- Boost the protein: Add grilled chicken, shrimp, or chickpeas for an extra protein boost.

APPROXIMATE NUTRITIONAL INFO (PER SERVING)

- Calories: 200
- Protein: 5g
- Fiber: 5g
- Healthy Fats: 15g
- Vitamin K: 100% Daily Value

LUNCH: FLAVORFUL AND FILLING GERD-FRIENDLY RECIPES
MEDITERRANEAN QUINOA BOWL

Prep time: 15 minutes (if quinoa is pre-cooked) | **Serving size: 2** | **Special considerations:** Gluten-free, vegetarian, high in fiber, customizable | **Budget-friendly tip:** Buy quinoa in bulk and cook a large batch to use throughout the week

Why It's a GERD-Friendly Winner

This vibrant bowl is a nutritional powerhouse, combining the complete protein of quinoa with a rainbow of fresh veggies, heart-healthy fats, and a zesty lemon-olive oil dressing. It's a light yet satisfying lunch that won't weigh you down or trigger your symptoms.

INGREDIENTS

- Salad:
  - 1 cup cooked quinoa
  - ½ cup chopped cucumber
  - ½ cup chopped tomato (seeded and drained)
  - ¼ cup Kalamata olives, pitted and halved
  - 2 tablespoons crumbled feta cheese (optional)
  - ¼ cup chopped red onion

- Lemon-Olive Oil Dressing:
  - 2 tablespoons extra-virgin olive oil
  - 1 tablespoon lemon juice
  - Pinch of salt, pepper, and dried oregano

INSTRUCTIONS

4. Combine Salad: In a large bowl, toss together the cooked quinoa, cucumber, tomato, olives, feta (if using), and red onion.
5. Make Dressing: In a small bowl, whisk together the olive oil, lemon juice, salt, pepper, and oregano.

6. Dress and Serve: Drizzle the dressing over the salad and toss gently to coat

TIPS

- Bulk it up: Add other GERD-friendly veggies like shredded carrots, chopped bell peppers, or diced zucchini.
- Flavor variation: Experiment with different Mediterranean herbs like basil or mint.
- Make-ahead meal: This salad keeps well in the refrigerator for up to 3 days, making it a great option for meal prepping.

APPROXIMATE NUTRITIONAL INFO (PER SERVING)

- Calories: 400
- Protein: 15g
- Fiber: 10g
- Healthy Fats: 25g
- Iron: 20% Daily Value

SESAME-CRUSTED CHICKEN & KALE SALAD

Prep time: 20 minutes | **Cook time:** 10 minutes | **Serving size:** 2 | **Special considerations:** Gluten-free, high in protein, customizable | **Budget-friendly tip**: If chicken breasts are too expensive, use boneless, skinless chicken thighs instead.

Why It's a GERD-Friendly Winner

This Asian-inspired salad is a protein powerhouse, thanks to the lean chicken breast and edamame. Kale provides a hearty base of fiber and nutrients, while toasted sesame seeds and a ginger-sesame dressing add a burst of flavor without relying on spicy ingredients.

INGREDIENTS

- Chicken:
    - 1 boneless, skinless chicken breast
    - 1 tablespoon sesame seeds
    - Salt and pepper to taste
- Salad:
    - 2 cups chopped kale, massaged with a squeeze of lemon juice
    - ½ cup cooked edamame (shelled)
    - ½ cup shredded carrots

- Sesame-Ginger Dressing:
    - 2 tablespoons low-sodium soy sauce (or tamari for gluten-free)
    - 1 tablespoon rice vinegar
    - 1 teaspoon grated fresh ginger
    - 1 teaspoon sesame oil
    - ½ teaspoon honey (optional)

INSTRUCTIONS

1. Prep the chicken: Pound the chicken breast to an even thickness. Season with salt and pepper. Press sesame seeds into both sides.
2. Cook the chicken: Heat a drizzle of olive oil in a skillet over medium heat. Cook the chicken for 4-5 minutes per side, or until cooked through. Let rest and then slice.

3. Massage the kale: In a large bowl, gently massage the kale with lemon juice to soften it.
4. Assemble the salad: Add the cooked edamame, shredded carrots, and sliced chicken to the kale.
5. Make the dressing: Whisk together soy sauce, rice vinegar, ginger, sesame oil, and honey (if using).
6. Dress and serve: Drizzle the dressing over the salad and toss to coat.

TIPS

- For a vegetarian option: Substitute the chicken for baked tofu or tempeh.
- Spice it up (if tolerated): Add a pinch of red pepper flakes to the dressing for a little heat.
- Nutty alternative: If sesame seeds are a trigger for you, use finely chopped walnuts or almonds for the crust.

APPROXIMATE NUTRITIONAL INFO (PER SERVING)

- Calories: 350
- Protein: 35g
- Fiber: 8g
- Healthy Fats: 15g
- Iron: 25% Daily Value

HERBED LENTIL & CUCUMBER SALAD

Prep time: 15 minutes (if lentils are pre-cooked) | **Serving size:** 2 | **Special considerations:** Vegan (omit feta), gluten-free, high in fiber, budget-friendly | **Budget-friendly tip:** Lentils are an inexpensive and nutritious pantry staple

Why It's a GERD-Friendly Winner

This light and refreshing salad is packed with protein, fiber, and fresh herbs. Lentils are a great plant-based protein source, and cucumbers and tomatoes add hydration and vitamins. The simple red wine vinegar dressing provides a tangy kick without the acidity of citrus.

INGREDIENTS

- Salad:
  - 1 cup cooked lentils
  - ½ cup chopped cucumber
  - ½ cup chopped tomatoes (seeded and drained)
  - 2 tablespoons chopped fresh dill
  - 2 tablespoons chopped fresh parsley
  - 2 tablespoons crumbled feta cheese (optional)

- Red Wine Vinegar Dressing:
  - 2 tablespoons red wine vinegar
  - 1 tablespoon olive oil
  - Pinch of salt, pepper, and dried oregano

INSTRUCTIONS

1. **Combine Salad:** In a bowl, combine cooked lentils, cucumber, tomatoes, dill, parsley, and feta (if using).
2. **Make Dressing:** In a small bowl, whisk together red wine vinegar, olive oil, salt, pepper, and oregano.
3. **Dress and Serve:** Pour the dressing over the salad and toss gently to coat.

TIPS

- Herb it up: Experiment with different fresh herbs like basil, mint, or cilantro.
- Add crunch: Sprinkle with sunflower seeds or chopped walnuts for extra texture.
- Make it ahead: This salad is perfect for meal prepping and keeps well in the refrigerator for up to 3 days.

APPROXIMATE NUTRITIONAL INFO (PER SERVING)

- Calories: 300
- Protein: 15g
- Fiber: 12g
- Healthy Fats: 12g
- Iron: 30% Daily Value

WATERMELON, FETA & MINT SALAD

Prep time: 10 minutes | **Chill time:** 30 minutes (optional) | **Serving size:** 2 | **Special considerations:** Vegetarian, gluten-free, low in calories, naturally sweet | **Budget-friendly tip:** Watermelon is most affordable when in season

Why It's a GERD-Friendly Winner

This refreshing salad is a burst of summery flavors and a hydrating oasis for your gut. Watermelon is incredibly hydrating and naturally alkaline, while feta adds a salty tang and mint offers a cooling touch.

INGREDIENTS

- 4 cups cubed watermelon
- ½ cup crumbled feta cheese
- ½ cup chopped fresh mint
- ½ cup chopped cucumber

INSTRUCTIONS

1. In a large bowl, gently toss together watermelon, feta, mint, and cucumber.
2. Refrigerate for at least 30 minutes to allow flavors to meld (optional).
3. Enjoy chilled!

TIPS

- Quality feta: Invest in a good quality feta for the best flavor and texture.
- Flavor exploration: If you can tolerate a little heat, add a pinch of red pepper flakes. For a briny twist, try a few chopped Kalamata olives.
- Sweetness boost (optional): If you prefer a sweeter salad, drizzle with a tiny amount of honey or balsamic glaze.

APPROXIMATE NUTRITIONAL INFO (PER SERVING)

- Calories: 150
- Protein: 5g
- Fiber: 2g
- Healthy Fats: 5g
- Vitamin C: 30% Daily Value

SPINACH & AVOCADO SALAD WITH WALNUT VINAIGRETTE

Prep time: 10 minutes | **Serving size:** 2 | **Special considerations:** Vegan (omit feta), gluten-free, high in fiber | **Budget-friendly tip:** Buy spinach in bulk and wash and store it for easy use throughout the week

Why It's a GERD-Friendly Winner

This salad is a nutrient powerhouse, packed with fiber-rich spinach, healthy fats from avocado, and protein and omega-3s from walnuts. The light vinaigrette is made with olive oil and apple cider vinegar, avoiding the acidity of other vinegars.

INGREDIENTS

- Salad:
    - 8 cups baby spinach
    - 1 avocado, diced
    - ½ cup chopped walnuts
- Walnut Vinaigrette:
    - ¼ cup olive oil
    - 2 tablespoons apple cider vinegar
    - 1 tablespoon chopped walnuts
    - 1 teaspoon Dijon mustard
    - Pinch of salt and pepper

INSTRUCTIONS

1. Make the dressing: In a small bowl, whisk together olive oil, vinegar, chopped walnuts, Dijon mustard, salt, and pepper.
2. Assemble the salad: In a large bowl, combine spinach, avocado, and walnuts.
3. Dress and serve: Drizzle the dressing over the salad and toss gently to coat.

- Get creative with veggies: Add other GERD-friendly vegetables like sliced bell peppers, cucumbers, or shredded carrots.
- Boost the protein: Top with grilled chicken or a poached egg white for a more filling meal.
- Make it your own: Experiment with different types of vinegar in the dressing, such as balsamic or champagne vinegar (in moderation).

APPROXIMATE NUTRITIONAL INFO (PER SERVING)

- Calories: 350
- Protein: 8g
- Fiber: 10g
- Healthy Fats: 30g
- Vitamin E: 30% Daily Value

CURRIED SWEET POTATO & CARROT SOUP WITH GINGER & CASHEW CREAM

Prep time: 15 minutes | **Cook time:** 30 minutes | **Serving size:** 4 | **Special considerations:** Vegan, gluten-free (check the label on your curry paste), dairy-free, budget-friendly, easily adaptable for dietary preferences | **Budget-friendly tip:** Sweet potatoes and carrots are affordable and readily available year-round. Cashews can be purchased in bulk to save money.

Why It's a GERD-Friendly Winner

This creamy and comforting soup is a symphony of flavors and textures, all while being gentle on your digestive system. Sweet potatoes and carrots are naturally sweet and alkaline, helping to balance stomach acid. Ginger adds a warm, soothing touch, while yellow curry paste offers subtle spice without being overly irritating. The cashew cream provides a luxurious texture without the fat and dairy that can trigger reflux.

INGREDIENTS

- 2 tablespoons olive oil
- 1 onion, chopped
- 2 cloves garlic, minced
- 1 tablespoon grated fresh ginger
- 1 teaspoon yellow curry paste (adjust to your spice tolerance)
- 2 large sweet potatoes, peeled and chopped
- 2 large carrots, peeled and chopped
- 4 cups vegetable broth
- ½ cup raw cashews, soaked in water for at least 2 hours
- Salt and pepper to taste
- Fresh cilantro for garnish (optional)

INSTRUCTIONS

1. Sauté: Heat olive oil in a large pot over medium heat. Add onion and cook until softened, about 5 minutes. Add garlic and ginger, cook for 1 minute more.
2. Spice it up: Stir in curry paste and cook for 30 seconds, stirring constantly.

3. Simmer: Add sweet potatoes, carrots, and vegetable broth. Bring to a boil, then reduce heat and simmer until the vegetables are very tender, about 20 minutes.

4. Make cashew cream: Drain and rinse the soaked cashews. Blend them with ½ cup of fresh water until completely smooth and creamy.

5. Blend: Use an immersion blender to puree the soup until smooth (or carefully transfer to a blender in batches).

6. Finish: Stir in the cashew cream. Season to taste with salt and pepper.

7. Serve: Ladle into bowls. Garnish with fresh cilantro if desired.

TIPS

- Spice level: Adjust the amount of curry paste to your preference. If you're sensitive to spice, start with ½ teaspoon and add more as desired.
- Add more veggies: Feel free to add other GERD-friendly vegetables like cauliflower, zucchini, or spinach.
- Make it richer: For an extra creamy texture, add a splash of coconut milk along with the cashew cream.
- Freeze for later: This soup freezes well for convenient future meals.

APPROXIMATE NUTRITIONAL INFO (PER SERVING)

- Calories: 300
- Protein: 8g
- Fiber: 10g
- Healthy Fats: 15g
- Vitamin A: 200% Daily Value

ROASTED GARLIC & CAULIFLOWER SOUP

Prep time: 15 minutes | **Cook time:** 45 minutes | **Serving size:** 4 | **Special considerations:** Vegan, gluten-free (check the label on your vegetable broth), dairy-free, budget-friendly, easily adaptable for dietary preferences | **Budget-friendly tip:** Cauliflower is often more affordable than other cruciferous vegetables like broccoli. Look for sales or buy a whole head and use the leftovers in other dishes

Why It's a GERD-Friendly Winner

This creamy and flavorful soup is a comforting classic. Roasting the cauliflower and garlic brings out their natural sweetness, while the cashew cream adds richness without the dairy that can trigger reflux. Chives provide a subtle oniony flavor without being overly pungent.

INGREDIENTS

- 1 head of cauliflower, cut into florets
- 1 head of garlic, cloves separated and peeled
- 2 tablespoons olive oil
- 4 cups vegetable broth (low-sodium)
- ¼ cup raw cashews, soaked in water for at least 2 hours
- Salt and pepper to taste
- 2 tablespoons chopped fresh chives

INSTRUCTIONS

1. Preheat oven to 425°F (220°C).
2. Roast: Toss cauliflower florets and garlic cloves with 1 tablespoon olive oil, salt, and pepper. Spread on a baking sheet and roast for 20-25 minutes, or until tender and lightly browned.

3. Sauté: While the cauliflower is roasting, heat the remaining olive oil in a large pot over medium heat. Add the roasted cauliflower and garlic to the pot.

4. Simmer: Pour in the vegetable broth and bring to a simmer. Cook for 5 minutes to allow the flavors to meld.

5. Blend: Carefully transfer the soup to a blender (or use an immersion blender) and puree until completely smooth.

6. Make cashew cream: Drain and rinse the soaked cashews. Blend them with ½ cup of fresh water until smooth and creamy.

7. Combine: Stir the cashew cream into the soup and season with salt and pepper to taste.

8. Serve: Ladle into bowls and garnish with chopped chives.

TIPS

- Spice it up: If you tolerate mild spices, add a pinch of ground nutmeg or cumin for an extra layer of flavor.

- Add crunch: Top with toasted pumpkin seeds or a swirl of your favorite non-dairy yogurt for added texture and richness.

- Make it a meal: Serve with a side of whole-grain bread or crackers for a more satisfying lunch.

- Freeze for later: This soup freezes beautifully, so make a double batch and enjoy it later.

APPROXIMATE NUTRITIONAL INFO (PER SERVING)

- Calories: 250
- Protein: 7g
- Fiber: 8g
- Healthy Fats: 15g
- Vitamin C: 80% Daily Value

HUMMUS & VEGGIE PINWHEELS

Prep time: 15 minutes | **Serving size:** 4 pinwheels (2 per serving) | **Special considerations:** Vegetarian, vegan, gluten-free (if using gluten-free tortillas), customizable | **Budget-friendly tip:** Hummus is a versatile and affordable ingredient. You can easily make your own or buy it pre-made

Why It's a GERD-Friendly Winner

These colorful pinwheels are a fun and portable lunch option. The hummus provides protein and fiber from chickpeas, while the fresh veggies offer vitamins, minerals, and a satisfying crunch. The whole-wheat tortillas are a good source of fiber and complex carbohydrates.

INGREDIENTS

- 4 medium whole-wheat tortillas
- ½ cup hummus (plain or flavored)
- 1 cup shredded carrots
- 1 cup baby spinach leaves
- ½ cucumber, thinly sliced

INSTRUCTIONS

1. Lay out the tortillas on a flat surface.
2. Spread a thin layer of hummus evenly over each tortilla, leaving a small border around the edges.
3. Top with shredded carrots, spinach leaves, and cucumber slices.
4. Roll up each tortilla tightly, starting from one end.
5. Slice each roll into 1-inch thick pinwheels.

- Variety is key: Experiment with different hummus flavors and vegetable combinations.

- Make them ahead: Prepare these pinwheels the night before for a grab-and-go lunch.

- Keep them fresh: Store the pinwheels in an airtight container in the refrigerator for up to 3 days.

APPROXIMATE NUTRITIONAL INFO (PER SERVING)

- Calories: 200

- Protein: 8g

- Fiber: 8g

- Healthy Fats: 5g

- Vitamin A: 100% Daily Value

GRILLED CHICKEN & PINEAPPLE-FREE SALSA WRAP

Prep time: 15 minutes | **Cook time:** 10 minutes | **Serving size:** 2 wraps | **Special considerations:** Gluten-free (if using gluten-free tortillas), high in protein | **Budget-friendly tip:** Chicken breast is a lean and affordable protein option. Buy in bulk and grill or bake several breasts at once for meal prepping.

Why It's a GERD-Friendly Winner

This flavorful wrap is packed with lean protein from grilled chicken and a refreshing pineapple-free salsa. The whole-wheat tortilla provides fiber, and avocado adds healthy fats for satiety. By omitting pineapple, this salsa avoids the acidity that can trigger reflux in some people.

INGREDIENTS

- Chicken:
    - 1 boneless, skinless chicken breast
    - Salt, pepper, and GERD-friendly spices (like cumin, coriander, paprika)
- Salsa:
    - 1 cup chopped tomatoes (seeded and drained)
    - ¼ cup chopped red onion
    - 2 tablespoons chopped cilantro
    - Juice of ½ lime
    - Salt and pepper to taste
- Toppings:
    - ½ avocado, sliced
    - 2 large whole-wheat tortillas

INSTRUCTIONS

1. Grill chicken: Season the chicken breast with salt, pepper, and spices. Grill over medium heat until cooked through (or bake in the oven). Let rest and then slice.

2. Make salsa: In a bowl, combine chopped tomatoes, red onion, cilantro, lime juice, salt, and pepper.

3. Assemble the wraps: Warm the tortillas slightly. Layer with sliced grilled chicken, salsa, and avocado slices. Roll tightly.

TIPS

- Spice it up (if tolerated): Add a pinch of chili powder or chipotle powder to the chicken seasoning for a smoky kick.
- Prep ahead: Grill the chicken and make the salsa in advance for a quick and easy lunch.
- Swap the protein: Substitute the chicken for grilled shrimp, baked tofu, or cooked lentils.

APPROXIMATE NUTRITIONAL INFO (PER SERVING)

- Calories: 400
- Protein: 30g
- Fiber: 10g
- Healthy Fats: 15g
- Vitamin C: 50% Daily Value

LENTIL & SAUERKRAUT WRAP

Prep time: 10 minutes (if using pre-cooked lentils) | **Serving size:** 2 wraps | **Special considerations:** Vegan, gluten-free (if using gluten-free tortillas), high in fiber | **Budget-friendly tip:** Lentils and sauerkraut are both inexpensive and nutritious pantry staples

Why It's a GERD-Friendly Winner

This hearty wrap is packed with gut-healthy ingredients. Lentils provide protein and fiber, while sauerkraut offers probiotics that can aid digestion. The mustard adds a tangy flavor without the spice that can trigger reflux.

INGREDIENTS

- 1 cup cooked lentils
- ½ cup sauerkraut, drained
- 2 tablespoons Dijon mustard (or other mild mustard)
- 2 large whole-wheat tortillas
- Optional: leafy greens like spinach or arugula

INSTRUCTIONS

1. In a small bowl, combine the lentils and sauerkraut.
2. Spread a thin layer of mustard on each tortilla.
3. Divide the lentil and sauerkraut mixture between the tortillas.
4. Add a handful of leafy greens if desired.
5. Roll up the tortillas tightly and enjoy!

TIPS

- Warm it up: For a warm wrap, lightly toast the tortillas in a dry skillet before adding the fillings.
- Flavor exploration: Add a sprinkle of caraway seeds or chopped fresh dill for an extra dimension of flavor.
- Prep ahead: Cook the lentils in advance and store them in the refrigerator for quick and easy assembly.

APPROXIMATE NUTRITIONAL INFO (PER SERVING)

- Calories: 300
- Protein: 15g
- Fiber: 15g
- Healthy Fats: 5g
- Iron: 30% Daily Value

HERB-CRUSTED SALMON WITH ASPARAGUS & WHITE BEAN PURÉE

Prep time: 10 minutes | **Cook time:** 25 minutes | **Serving size:** 2 | **Special considerations:** Gluten-free, dairy-free, high in protein | **Budget-friendly tip:** Salmon can be pricey. Look for sales or consider less expensive fish like cod or tilapia. Canned cannellini beans are an economical pantry staple.

Why It's a GERD-Friendly Winner

This elegant dish is packed with nutrients and gentle on your stomach. Salmon, a lean protein, is rich in omega-3 fatty acids, which have anti-inflammatory properties. Asparagus provides fiber and vitamins, while the white bean purée offers a creamy base without the dairy that can trigger reflux. The herb crust adds a bright, fresh flavor without relying on harsh spices.

INGREDIENTS

- Salmon:
    - Two 6-ounce salmon fillets
    - 1 tablespoon chopped fresh dill
    - 1 tablespoon chopped fresh parsley
    - Zest of ½ lemon
    - Salt and pepper to taste
- Asparagus:
    - 1 bunch asparagus, trimmed
    - 1 teaspoon olive oil
- White Bean Purée:
    - ½ cup canned cannellini beans, rinsed and drained
    - 1 tablespoon lemon juice
    - 1 tablespoon olive oil
    - Salt and pepper to taste

INSTRUCTIONS

1. Preheat oven to 400°F (200°C).
2. Prepare salmon: Pat salmon fillets dry. In a small bowl, combine dill, parsley, lemon zest, salt, and pepper. Press herb mixture onto the top of each fillet.

3. Roast asparagus: Toss asparagus with olive oil, salt, and pepper. Spread on a baking sheet.

4. Bake: Place the salmon fillets on the same baking sheet with the asparagus. Bake for 10-12 minutes.

5. Make purée: While the salmon and asparagus roast, combine cannellini beans, lemon juice, and olive oil in a food processor or blender. Blend until smooth, adding a splash of water if needed to reach desired consistency. Season with salt and pepper.

6. Serve: Spread white bean purée on each plate, top with a salmon fillet and roasted asparagus.

TIPS

- Fish swap: Use cod, tilapia, or another white fish instead of salmon.
- Flavor variations: Try different herbs for the crust, such as thyme, rosemary, or a mix of your favorites.
- Make it creamy: Stir in a dollop of non-dairy yogurt or a drizzle of olive oil into the white bean purée for extra richness.

APPROXIMATE NUTRITIONAL INFO (PER SERVING)

- Calories: 450
- Protein: 35g
- Fiber: 10g
- Healthy Fats: 30g
- Vitamin C: 50% Daily Value

CHICKEN & QUINOA STUFFED PEPPERS

Prep time: 15 minutes | **Cook time:** 30 minutes | **Serving size:** 2 | **Special considerations:** Gluten-free, high in protein, customizable | **Budget-friendly tip:** Bell peppers are often in season and affordable during the summer months. You can also use ground turkey or lean ground beef instead of chicken.

Why It's a GERD-Friendly Winner

These colorful stuffed peppers are a fun and nutritious way to enjoy a balanced meal. The bell peppers provide fiber and vitamins, while the quinoa and chicken offer protein and complex carbohydrates. The filling is seasoned with onion and a touch of low-acid tomato sauce for flavor.

INGREDIENTS

- 2 bell peppers (any color), halved lengthwise and seeds removed
- ½ cup cooked quinoa
- ½ pound ground chicken
- ¼ cup chopped onion
- ¼ cup low-acid tomato sauce
- ¼ cup shredded mozzarella cheese (optional)
- Salt and pepper to taste
- Fresh herbs for garnish (optional)

INSTRUCTIONS

1. Preheat oven to 375°F (190°C).
2. Cook filling: In a skillet over medium heat, cook the ground chicken and onion until the chicken is browned and cooked through. Drain any excess fat.

3. Mix and stuff: Stir in the cooked quinoa, tomato sauce, salt, and pepper. Fill each bell pepper half with the mixture.

4. Bake: Place the stuffed peppers in a baking dish and bake for 20-25 minutes, or until the peppers are tender and the filling is heated through.

5. Add cheese (optional): If desired, sprinkle with mozzarella cheese during the last 5 minutes of baking.

6. Garnish and serve: Top with chopped fresh herbs like basil or parsley, if desired.

TIPS

- Veggie boost: Add other chopped vegetables like zucchini, mushrooms, or spinach to the filling.

- Vegetarian option: Substitute the ground chicken with lentils or crumbled tofu.

- Make ahead: Prepare the filling in advance and refrigerate. Stuff and bake the peppers just before serving.

APPROXIMATE NUTRITIONAL INFO (PER SERVING)

- Calories: 300
- Protein: 25g
- Fiber: 6g
- Healthy Fats: 10g
- Vitamin C: 150% Daily Value

SHRIMP & AVOCADO SALAD WITH LIME-CILANTRO DRESSING

Prep time: 15 minutes | **Serving size:** 2 | **Special considerations:** Gluten-free, dairy-free, high in protein | **Budget-friendly tip:** Buy frozen shrimp and thaw it overnight in the refrigerator to save money

Why It's a GERD-Friendly Winner

This light and refreshing salad is perfect for warmer days. Shrimp is a lean protein that's easy to digest, while avocado adds healthy fats and a creamy texture. The cucumber provides hydration and a cool crunch, and the cilantro lime dressing offers a bright and zesty flavor.

INGREDIENTS

- Salad:
  - 1 pound cooked shrimp, peeled and deveined
  - 1 avocado, diced
  - 1 cucumber, diced
  - ¼ cup chopped fresh cilantro

- Lime-Cilantro Dressing:
  - 2 tablespoons olive oil
  - Juice of 1 lime
  - 2 tablespoons chopped fresh cilantro
  - Salt and pepper to taste

INSTRUCTIONS

1. Make dressing: In a small bowl, whisk together olive oil, lime juice, cilantro, salt, and pepper.
2. Combine salad: In a large bowl, combine shrimp, avocado, cucumber, and cilantro.
3. Dress and serve: Pour the dressing over the salad and toss gently to coat. Serve immediately or chill for later.

TIPS

- Spice it up (if tolerated): Add a pinch of red pepper flakes to the dressing for a little heat.

- Add greens: Toss the salad with a bed of leafy greens like spinach or romaine for extra nutrients and fiber.

- Make ahead: The dressing can be prepared in advance and stored in the refrigerator for up to a week.

APPROXIMATE NUTRITIONAL INFO (PER SERVING)

- Calories: 350
- Protein: 30g
- Fiber: 8g
- Healthy Fats: 25g
- Vitamin C: 30% Daily Value

MUSHROOM & SPINACH QUINOA

Prep time: 10 minutes | **Cook time:** 15 minutes | **Serving size:** 2 | **Special considerations:** Vegan, gluten-free, high in fiber | **Budget-friendly tip:** Buy mushrooms in bulk and freeze them for later use. Quinoa is also a cost-effective grain that can be cooked in large batches for meal prepping

Why It's a GERD-Friendly Winner

This simple yet satisfying dish is packed with nutrients and flavor. Quinoa is a complete protein that's also high in fiber and gentle on digestion. Mushrooms provide umami flavor and vitamins, while spinach adds a boost of iron and other essential nutrients.

INGREDIENTS

- 1 cup cooked quinoa

- 1 tablespoon olive oil

- 1 cup sliced mushrooms

- 1 cup baby spinach

- 1 cup vegetable broth (low-sodium)

- ¼ teaspoon garlic powder

- Pinch of dried thyme

- Salt and pepper to taste

INSTRUCTIONS

1. Sauté: Heat olive oil in a large skillet over medium heat. Add mushrooms and cook until softened and lightly browned, about 5-7 minutes.
2. Wilt spinach: Add spinach and cook until wilted, about 1 minute.
3. Simmer: Stir in cooked quinoa, vegetable broth, garlic powder, thyme, salt, and pepper. Bring to a simmer and cook until most of the liquid is absorbed, about 5 minutes.
4. Serve: Taste and adjust seasoning with salt and pepper as needed. Serve warm.

- Calories: 300
- Protein: 10g
- Fiber: 8g
- Healthy Fats: 10g
- Iron: 30% Daily Value
- Vitamin A: 20% Daily Value
- Vitamin C: 25% Daily Value
- Potassium: 15% Daily Value

DINNER: FLAVORFUL & SATISFYING GERD-FRIENDLY RECIPES

GINGER-GLAZED SALMON WITH ROASTED VEGETABLES

Prep time: 15 minutes | **Cook time:** 25-30 minutes | **Serving size:** 2 | **Special considerations:** Gluten-free, dairy-free, high in protein and omega-3s | **Budget-friendly tip:** Salmon can be pricey. Look for sales or try a less expensive fish like cod or tilapia. Frozen vegetables can be a more economical option than fresh.

Why It's a GERD-Friendly Winner

This dish is a symphony of flavors and textures, featuring the omega-3-rich salmon glazed with a soothing ginger-honey mixture and roasted alongside a colorful medley of vegetables. The sweetness of the glaze balances the savory fish, while the roasted vegetables provide fiber and nutrients.

INGREDIENTS

- Salmon:
    - Two 6-ounce salmon fillets
    - 1 tablespoon grated fresh ginger
    - 1 tablespoon low-sodium soy sauce (or tamari for gluten-free)
    - 1 tablespoon honey

- Roasted Vegetables:
    - 1 head broccoli, cut into florets
    - 2 carrots, peeled and chopped
    - 1 sweet potato, peeled and cubed
    - 1 tablespoon olive oil
    - Salt and pepper to taste

INSTRUCTIONS

1. Preheat oven to 400°F (200°C).
2. Prepare salmon: In a small bowl, whisk together ginger, soy sauce (or tamari), and honey. Place salmon fillets on a baking sheet lined with parchment paper. Brush the glaze generously over the salmon.

3. Roast vegetables: In a separate bowl, toss broccoli, carrots, and sweet potato with olive oil, salt, and pepper. Spread the vegetables on the baking sheet around the salmon.

4. Bake: Roast for 25-30 minutes, or until the salmon is cooked through and the vegetables are tender.

TIPS

- Ginger variation: If you're not a fan of ginger, try using a different herb or spice in the glaze, such as garlic, dill, or paprika.

- Vegetable swap: Feel free to substitute your favorite GERD-friendly vegetables for the broccoli, carrots, and sweet potatoes.

- Serving suggestion: Serve the salmon and roasted vegetables over a bed of brown rice or quinoa for a complete meal.

APPROXIMATE NUTRITIONAL INFO (PER SERVING)

- Calories: 450
- Protein: 35g
- Fiber: 10g
- Healthy Fats: 20g
- Omega-3 Fatty Acids: 2000mg

CHICKEN & VEGGIE COCONUT CURRY

Prep time: 15 minutes | **Cook time:** 25-30 minutes | **Serving size**: 4 | **Special considerations:** Gluten-free, dairy-free, high in protein | **Budget-friendly tip:** Use canned coconut milk instead of carton coconut milk for a more affordable option. You can also substitute chicken thighs for breasts.

Why It's a GERD-Friendly Winner

This creamy curry is packed with flavor and gentle on your stomach. Lean chicken breast provides protein, while the array of vegetables offers fiber and nutrients. The coconut milk base is a soothing alternative to dairy, and the turmeric, ginger, and curry powder provide warm, anti-inflammatory spices without being overly irritating.

INGREDIENTS

- 1 tablespoon olive oil
- 1 onion, chopped
- 2 bell peppers (any color), chopped
- 1 head cauliflower, cut into florets
- 1 pound boneless, skinless chicken breasts, cut into bite-sized pieces
- 1 tablespoon grated fresh ginger
- 1 teaspoon turmeric powder
- ½ teaspoon curry powder
- 1 (14-ounce) can light coconut milk
- Salt and pepper to taste
- Cooked brown rice for serving

INSTRUCTIONS

1. Heat olive oil in a large pot or Dutch oven over medium heat. Add onion and cook until softened, about 5 minutes.
2. Add bell peppers and cauliflower and cook for 5 minutes more.
3. Add chicken, ginger, turmeric, and curry powder. Cook, stirring occasionally, until chicken is cooked through, about 5-7 minutes.
4. Stir in coconut milk and bring to a simmer. Cook for 10-15 minutes, or until the vegetables are tender and the sauce has thickened slightly.
5. Season with salt and pepper to taste.

6. Serve over brown rice.

TIPS

- Spice it up (if tolerated): Add a pinch of cayenne pepper for a touch of heat.
- Veggie variations: Feel free to swap in your favorite GERD-friendly vegetables, such as broccoli, carrots, or sweet potatoes.
- Make it vegetarian: Omit the chicken and add extra vegetables or chickpeas for a plant-based meal.

APPROXIMATE NUTRITIONAL INFO (PER SERVING)

- Calories: 300
- Protein: 15g
- Fiber: 12g
- Healthy Fats: 12g
- Iron: 30% Daily Value

SHRIMP & AVOCADO QUINOA BOWLS

Prep time: 10 minutes | **Cook time:** 15 minutes | **Serving size:** 2 | **Special considerations:** Gluten-free, dairy-free, high in protein | **Budget-friendly tip**: Frozen shrimp is often more affordable than fresh. You can also use pre-cooked quinoa to save time.

Why It's a GERD-Friendly Winner

This light and refreshing bowl is packed with lean protein from shrimp, complex carbohydrates from quinoa, and healthy fats from avocado. The garlic, lime juice, and chili powder add a zesty flavor without being overly spicy.

INGREDIENTS

- 1 pound shrimp, peeled and deveined
- 1 tablespoon olive oil
- 2 cloves garlic, minced
- Juice of 1 lime
- ½ teaspoon chili powder
- Salt and pepper to taste
- 1 cup cooked quinoa
- 1 avocado, diced
- ½ cup chopped cucumber
- ¼ cup chopped fresh cilantro
- Lime wedges for serving

INSTRUCTIONS

1. Heat olive oil in a large skillet over medium heat. Add shrimp and cook until pink and opaque, about 3-4 minutes per side.

2. Add garlic, lime juice, chili powder, salt, and pepper to the skillet. Cook for 1 minute more, or until fragrant.

3. Divide the quinoa between two bowls. Top with shrimp, avocado, cucumber, and cilantro.

4. Squeeze a lime wedge over each bowl and serve.

TIPS

- Spice it up (if tolerated): Add a pinch of cayenne pepper for extra heat.
- Veggie variations: Feel free to swap in your favorite GERD-friendly vegetables, such as chopped bell peppers or cherry tomatoes.
- Make it a meal prep: Prepare the quinoa and shrimp in advance for a quick and easy lunch or dinner.

APPROXIMATE NUTRITIONAL INFO (PER SERVING)

- Calories: 450
- Protein: 30g
- Fiber: 10g
- Healthy Fats: 20g

MEDITERRANEAN BAKED FISH

Prep time: 10 minutes | **Cook time**: 20 minutes | **Serving size: 2** | **Special considerations:** Gluten-free, dairy-free, low in fat | **Budget-friendly tip:** Cod and tilapia are often more affordable than other types of fish.

Why It's a GERD-Friendly Winner

This simple yet elegant dish is a flavorful and healthy option for those with GERD. White fish like cod or tilapia is a lean protein source, and the tomatoes, olives, and capers add a burst of Mediterranean flavor. Baking the fish in parchment paper helps retain moisture and ensures gentle cooking.

INGREDIENTS

- Two 6-ounce white fish fillets (cod, tilapia, or other)
- 1 cup cherry tomatoes, halved
- ¼ cup Kalamata olives, pitted and halved
- 1 tablespoon capers, drained
- 1 lemon, sliced
- 1 tablespoon olive oil
- ½ teaspoon dried oregano
- Salt and pepper to taste
- 2 sheets parchment paper

INSTRUCTIONS

1. Preheat oven to 400°F (200°C).
2. Fold each sheet of parchment paper in half. Place a fish fillet on one half of each sheet.

3. Top each fillet with half of the tomatoes, olives, capers, lemon slices, olive oil, oregano, salt, and pepper.

4. Fold the other half of the parchment paper over the fish and crimp the edges to seal.

5. Place the packets on a baking sheet and bake for 20 minutes, or until the fish is cooked through.

6. Open the packets carefully (watch for steam) and serve.

TIPS

- Spice it up (if tolerated): Add a pinch of red pepper flakes for a little heat, if you can handle it.
- Herb variations: Experiment with different herbs like basil, thyme, or rosemary.
- Make it a meal: Serve with a side of brown rice or a simple salad for a complete and satisfying dinner.

APPROXIMATE NUTRITIONAL INFO (PER SERVING)

- Calories: 300
- Protein: 30g
- Fiber: 4g
- Healthy Fats: 12g
- Vitamin C: 40% Daily Value
- Vitamin D: 60% Daily Value (depending on the type of fish)

ROASTED BUTTERNUT SQUASH & LENTIL SOUP WITH CURRY & WALNUT YOGURT SWIRL

Prep time: 15 minutes | **Cook time:** 45-50 minutes | **Serving size**: 4 | **Special considerations:** Vegan, gluten-free (ensure curry powder is gluten-free), dairy-free | **Budget-friendly tip:** Butternut squash is a winter squash and is most affordable during the fall and winter months. You can also use canned pumpkin puree instead for a budget-friendly alternative.

Why It's a GERD-Friendly Winner

This velvety soup is both comforting and nourishing. Roasted butternut squash adds natural sweetness and a creamy texture, while lentils provide protein and fiber to keep you satisfied. Curry powder offers a hint of warmth and depth, and the walnut yogurt swirl adds a touch of tangy richness without the fat and dairy that can trigger reflux.

INGREDIENTS

- 1 medium butternut squash, peeled, seeded, and cubed
- 1 tablespoon olive oil
- 1 onion, chopped
- 2 cloves garlic, minced
- 1 teaspoon curry powder
- ½ teaspoon ground cumin
- 1 cup red lentils, rinsed
- 4 cups vegetable broth (low-sodium)
- ½ cup plain plant-based yogurt
- ¼ cup chopped walnuts
- Salt and pepper to taste

INSTRUCTIONS

1. Preheat oven to 400°F (200°C).
2. Roast squash: Toss butternut squash cubes with olive oil, salt, and pepper. Spread on a baking sheet and roast for 25-30 minutes, or until tender.
3. Sauté: While the squash is roasting, heat olive oil in a large pot over medium heat. Add onion and cook until softened, about 5 minutes. Add garlic, curry powder, and cumin; cook for 1 minute more.

4. Simmer: Add roasted squash, lentils, and vegetable broth to the pot. Bring to a boil, then reduce heat and simmer for 15-20 minutes, or until the lentils are tender.

5. Blend: Use an immersion blender to puree the soup until smooth (or carefully transfer to a blender in batches).

6. Serve: Ladle the soup into bowls. Top each bowl with a dollop of yogurt and a sprinkle of walnuts.

TIPS

- Spice level: Adjust the amount of curry powder to your preference.
- Vegan yogurt: Choose your favorite plant-based yogurt for the topping.
- Add greens: Stir in a handful of spinach or kale at the end of cooking for extra nutrients.

APPROXIMATE NUTRITIONAL INFO (PER SERVING)

- Calories: 350
- Protein: 15g
- Fiber: 12g
- Healthy Fats: 18g

\

LEMONY HERB CHICKEN WITH ASPARAGUS & ZUCCHINI

Prep time: 10 minutes | **Cook time:** 25-30 minutes | **Serving size:** 2 | **Special considerations:** Gluten-free, dairy-free, high in protein | **Budget-friendly tip:** Boneless, skinless chicken breasts are often on sale. You can also use bone-in chicken breasts, which are usually less expensive, but be sure to adjust the cooking time accordingly.

Why It's a GERD-Friendly Winner

This simple yet flavorful dish features baked chicken breast seasoned with lemon, thyme, and rosemary – herbs known for their soothing properties. Asparagus and zucchini are low-acid vegetables that provide fiber and antioxidants. Quinoa, a gluten-free grain, offers complex carbohydrates and protein for a balanced meal.

INGREDIENTS

- 2 boneless, skinless chicken breasts
- 1 lemon, zested and juiced
- 1 teaspoon dried thyme
- 1 teaspoon dried rosemary
- Salt and pepper to taste
- 1 bunch asparagus, trimmed
- 2 medium zucchini, sliced
- 1 tablespoon olive oil
- Cooked quinoa for serving

INSTRUCTIONS

1. Preheat oven to 400°F (200°C).
2. Prepare chicken: In a small bowl, combine lemon zest, lemon juice, thyme, rosemary, salt, and pepper. Rub the mixture all over the chicken breasts.

3. Assemble: Place the chicken breasts on a baking sheet lined with parchment paper. Arrange asparagus and zucchini around the chicken. Drizzle vegetables with olive oil and season with salt and pepper.
4. Bake: Bake for 25-30 minutes, or until the chicken is cooked through and the vegetables are tender.
5. Serve: Plate the chicken and vegetables over a bed of cooked quinoa.

TIPS

- Herb variations: Feel free to use your favorite fresh or dried herbs, such as dill, oregano, or basil.
- Make it ahead: The chicken and vegetables can be prepared and assembled the night before. Simply bake when ready to eat.

APPROXIMATE NUTRITIONAL INFO (PER SERVING)

- Calories: 400
- Protein: 40g
- Fiber: 10g
- Healthy Fats: 15g

HERBED LENTIL & CUCUMBER SALAD

Prep time: 15 minutes (if lentils are pre-cooked) | **Serving size:** 2 | **Special considerations:** Vegan (omit feta), gluten-free, high in fiber, budget-friendly | **Budget-friendly tip:** Lentils are an inexpensive and nutritious pantry staple

Why It's a GERD-Friendly Winner

This light and refreshing salad is packed with protein, fiber, and fresh herbs. Lentils are a great plant-based protein source, and cucumbers and tomatoes add hydration and vitamins. The simple red wine vinegar dressing provides a tangy kick without the acidity of citrus.

INGREDIENTS

- Salad:
  - 1 cup cooked lentils
  - ½ cup chopped cucumber
  - ½ cup chopped tomatoes (seeded and drained)
  - 2 tablespoons chopped fresh dill
  - 2 tablespoons chopped fresh parsley
  - 2 tablespoons crumbled feta cheese (optional)

- Red Wine Vinegar Dressing:
  - 2 tablespoons red wine vinegar
  - 1 tablespoon olive oil
  - Pinch of salt, pepper, and dried oregano

INSTRUCTIONS

4. **Combine Salad:** In a bowl, combine cooked lentils, cucumber, tomatoes, dill, parsley, and feta (if using).
5. **Make Dressing:** In a small bowl, whisk together red wine vinegar, olive oil, salt, pepper, and oregano.
6. **Dress and Serve:** Pour the dressing over the salad and toss gently to coat.

- Herb it up: Experiment with different fresh herbs like basil, mint, or cilantro.

- Add crunch: Sprinkle with sunflower seeds or chopped walnuts for extra texture.

- Make it ahead: This salad is perfect for meal prepping and keeps well in the refrigerator for up to 3 days.

APPROXIMATE NUTRITIONAL INFO (PER SERVING)

- Calories: 300
- Protein: 15g
- Fiber: 12g
- Healthy Fats: 12g
- Iron: 30% Daily Value

TOFU SCRAMBLE WITH SPINACH & MUSHROOMS

Prep time: 10 minutes | **Cook time:** 15 minutes | **Serving size:** 2 | **Special considerations:** Vegan, gluten-free, high in protein | **Budget-friendly tip:** Tofu is an affordable and versatile plant-based protein source. Buy extra-firm tofu and press it to remove excess water before cooking.

Why It's a GERD-Friendly Winner

This vegan scramble is a hearty and satisfying meal that's easy on the digestive system. Crumbled tofu provides protein and a texture similar to scrambled eggs, while spinach and mushrooms offer fiber and nutrients. Turmeric adds a vibrant color and anti-inflammatory benefits, and nutritional yeast provides a cheesy flavor without the dairy.

INGREDIENTS

- 1 block extra-firm tofu, drained and crumbled
- 1 tablespoon olive oil
- 1 onion, chopped
- 2 cups sliced mushrooms
- 2 cups baby spinach
- 1 teaspoon turmeric powder
- 2 tablespoons nutritional yeast
- Salt and pepper to taste
- Roasted potato cubes for serving

INSTRUCTIONS

1. Heat olive oil in a large skillet over medium heat. Add onion and cook until softened, about 5 minutes.
2. Add mushrooms and cook until softened and lightly browned, about 5-7 minutes.
3. Add crumbled tofu and turmeric powder. Cook, stirring occasionally, until heated through, about 5 minutes.
4. Stir in spinach and cook until wilted, about 1 minute.
5. Remove from heat and stir in nutritional yeast, salt, and pepper.
6. Serve warm with roasted potato cubes.

- Spice it up: Add a pinch of red pepper flakes or chili powder for a little heat.

- Veggie variations: Try different vegetables like chopped broccoli, bell peppers, or kale.

- Make it a wrap: Fill tortillas with the scramble, avocado slices, and a drizzle of your favorite GERD-friendly sauce.

APPROXIMATE NUTRITIONAL INFO (PER SERVING)

- Calories: 350
- Protein: 20g
- Fiber: 12g
- Healthy Fats: 15g

STUFFED BELL PEPPERS WITH GROUND TURKEY, RICE, & SPINACH

Prep time: 15 minutes | **Cook time:** 45 minutes | **Serving size**: 4 | **Special considerations:** Gluten-free, dairy-free (omit cheese), high in **protein** | **Budget-friendly tip:** Ground turkey is a lean and affordable protein option. Choose bell peppers that are in season for the best price and flavor.

Why It's a GERD-Friendly Winner

These colorful stuffed peppers are a delicious and healthy way to enjoy a balanced meal. Bell peppers are packed with vitamins and fiber, while ground turkey and brown rice provide protein and complex carbohydrates. The spinach adds a boost of iron and other nutrients, and a small amount of tomato sauce provides flavor without too much acidity.

INGREDIENTS

- 4 bell peppers (any color), halved lengthwise and seeds removed
- 1 tablespoon olive oil
- 1 onion, chopped
- 1 pound ground turkey
- 1 cup cooked brown rice
- 1 cup chopped spinach
- ¼ cup low-acid tomato sauce
- ½ cup crumbled feta cheese (optional)
- Salt and pepper to taste
- Fresh herbs for garnish (optional)

INSTRUCTIONS

1. Preheat oven to 375°F (190°C).
2. Cook filling: Heat olive oil in a large skillet over medium heat. Add onion and cook until softened, about 5 minutes. Add ground turkey and cook until browned and cooked through. Drain any excess fat.
3. Combine ingredients: Stir in cooked rice, spinach, tomato sauce, salt, and pepper.
4. Stuff peppers: Fill each bell pepper half with the mixture.
5. Bake: Place the stuffed peppers in a baking dish and bake for

6. 45 minutes, or until the peppers are tender and the filling is heated through.

7. Add cheese (optional): If desired, sprinkle with feta cheese during the last 5 minutes of baking.

8. Garnish and serve: Top with chopped fresh herbs like basil or parsley, if desired.

TIPS

- Veggie variations: Add other chopped vegetables like zucchini, mushrooms, or corn to the filling.
- Dairy-free option: Omit the feta cheese or use a dairy-free alternative like vegan cheese or nutritional yeast.
- Make ahead: Prepare the filling in advance and refrigerate. Stuff and bake the peppers just before serving.

APPROXIMATE NUTRITIONAL INFO (PER SERVING)

- Calories: 350
- Protein: 28g
- Fiber: 7g
- Healthy Fats: 12g
- Vitamin C: 150% Daily Value

SWEET POTATO BLACK BEAN BURGERS ON LETTUCE WRAPS

Prep time: 20 minutes | **Cook time:** 20-25 minutes (baking) or 10-12 minutes (pan-frying) | **Serving size:** 4 burgers | **Special considerations:** Vegan, gluten-free, high in fiber, customizable | **Budget-friendly tip:** Sweet potatoes and black beans are affordable pantry staples. Look for sales on lettuce or grow your own.

Why It's a GERD-Friendly Winner

These flavorful veggie burgers are a delicious and satisfying alternative to traditional beef burgers. Sweet potatoes offer a naturally sweet and fiber-rich base, while black beans provide plant-based protein and iron. The lettuce wraps eliminate the gluten and potential heartburn triggers of bread buns.

INGREDIENTS

- Burgers:
    - 1 large sweet potato, peeled and cubed
    - 1 (15-ounce) can black beans, rinsed and drained
    - ½ cup chopped onion
    - ½ cup rolled oats (or breadcrumbs for gluten-free option)
    - 1 tablespoon chili powder
    - 1 teaspoon cumin
    - ½ teaspoon garlic powder
    - Salt and pepper to taste
- Toppings:
    - Avocado slices
    - Dijon mustard (or your preferred mustard)
    - Lettuce leaves (butter lettuce or romaine)

INSTRUCTIONS

1. **Cook sweet potato:** Boil or steam the sweet potato cubes until tender. Drain and mash.
2. **Mash beans:** Mash the black beans with a fork or potato masher.

3. **Combine ingredients:** In a large bowl, combine the mashed sweet potato, mashed black beans, onion, oats (or breadcrumbs), chili powder, cumin, garlic powder, salt, and pepper. Mix well.

4. **Form patties:** Divide the mixture into 4 equal portions and shape into patties.

5. **Bake or pan-fry:**

   - **Bake:** Place the patties on a baking sheet lined with parchment paper. Bake at 375°F (190°C) for 20-25 minutes, flipping halfway through.

   - **Pan-fry:** Heat a drizzle of olive oil in a skillet over medium heat. Cook the patties for 5-6 minutes per side, or until golden brown and cooked through.

6. **Assemble:** Place each patty on a lettuce leaf. Top with avocado slices and mustard.

TIPS

- Spice it up (if tolerated): Add a pinch of cayenne pepper or a dash of hot sauce to the burger mixture for a little kick.
- Make them ahead: The burgers can be formed and refrigerated or frozen for later use.
- Serving suggestions: Enjoy these burgers with a side salad or a cup of GERD-friendly soup.

APPROXIMATE NUTRITIONAL INFO (PER SERVING)

- Calories: 300
- Protein: 12g
- Fiber: 10g
- Healthy Fats: 8g

HERBED QUINOA & WHITE BEAN SALAD

Prep time: 15 minutes | **Serving size:** 2 | **Special considerations:** Vegan, gluten-free, high in fiber | **Budget-friendly tip:** Quinoa and cannellini beans are affordable pantry staples. Use seasonal herbs for the best flavor and value.

Why It's a GERD-Friendly Winner

This light and refreshing salad is packed with protein, fiber, and fresh herbs, making it a satisfying and gut-friendly meal. Quinoa provides all the essential amino acids, while cannellini beans offer additional protein and fiber. The cucumber and herbs add a cool, crisp element, and the lemon-olive oil dressing provides a bright and flavorful finish.

INGREDIENTS

- Salad:
    - 1 cup cooked quinoa
    - 1 (15-ounce) can cannellini beans, rinsed and drained
    - ½ cup chopped cucumber
    - 2 tablespoons chopped fresh dill
    - 2 tablespoons chopped fresh parsley

- Lemon-Olive Oil Dressing:
    - 2 tablespoons extra-virgin olive oil
    - 1 tablespoon lemon juice
    - Pinch of salt and pepper

INSTRUCTIONS

1. **Combine salad:** In a large bowl, combine cooked quinoa, cannellini beans, cucumber, dill, and parsley.
2. **Make dressing:** In a small bowl, whisk together olive oil, lemon juice, salt, and pepper.
3. **Dress and serve:** Pour the dressing over the salad and toss to coat.

- Add more veggies: For extra flavor and nutrients, add other GERD-friendly vegetables like chopped bell peppers, cherry tomatoes, or avocado.
- Make it a meal: Top the salad with grilled chicken or fish for additional protein.
- Prep ahead: This salad can be made ahead of time and stored in the refrigerator for up to 3 days.

APPROXIMATE NUTRITIONAL INFO (PER SERVING)

- Calories: 350
- Protein: 18g
- Fiber: 15g
- Healthy Fats: 12g

HONEY-ROASTED CARROTS & PARSNIPS

Prep time: 10 minutes | **Cook time:** 30-35 minutes | **Serving size:** 4 | **Special considerations:** Vegan, gluten-free, naturally sweet | **Budget-friendly tip:** Carrots and parsnips are both affordable root vegetables that are readily available year-round.

Why It's a GERD-Friendly Winner

This simple side dish is packed with flavor and nutrients. Carrots and parsnips are naturally sweet and high in fiber, while honey adds a touch of sweetness without being overly acidic. Olive oil and thyme enhance the flavors and provide a subtle earthy aroma.

INGREDIENTS

- 2 large carrots, peeled and chopped
- 2 parsnips, peeled and chopped
- 2 tablespoons olive oil
- 2 tablespoons honey
- 1 teaspoon dried thyme
- Salt and pepper to taste

INSTRUCTIONS

1. Preheat oven to 400°F (200°C).
2. Toss: In a large bowl, combine carrots, parsnips, olive oil, honey, thyme, salt, and pepper. Toss to coat evenly.
3. Roast: Spread the vegetables in a single layer on a baking sheet lined with parchment paper. Roast for 30-35 minutes, or until tender and caramelized, stirring occasionally.

TIPS

- Honey substitute: If you prefer a less sweet dish, use maple syrup or agave nectar instead of honey.
- Herb variations: Experiment with different herbs like rosemary or sage.
- Add some spice: A pinch of cayenne pepper can add a subtle kick.

APPROXIMATE NUTRITIONAL INFO (PER SERVING)

- Calories: 150
- Fiber: 5g
- Sugars: 10g (from honey)

GARLIC-SESAME GREEN BEANS

Prep time: 5 minutes | **Cook time:** 5-7 minutes | **Serving size:** 4 | **Special considerations:** Vegan, gluten-free (if using tamari instead of soy sauce) | **Budget-friendly tip:** Green beans are an affordable and versatile vegetable. Look for them on sale or buy them frozen to save money.

Why It's a GERD-Friendly Winner

These flavorful green beans are a quick and easy side dish. Steaming the beans helps retain their nutrients, while the garlic and sesame oil add a savory depth of flavor. A touch of soy sauce (or tamari) provides umami without being overly salty.

INGREDIENTS

- 1 pound green beans, trimmed
- 1 tablespoon sesame oil
- 2 cloves garlic, minced
- 1 tablespoon low-sodium soy sauce (or tamari)
- Pinch of red pepper flakes (optional)
- Sesame seeds for garnish (optional)

INSTRUCTIONS

1. **Steam:** Steam the green beans until tender-crisp, about 5-7 minutes.
2. **Sauté:** While the beans are steaming, heat the sesame oil in a small skillet over medium heat. Add garlic and cook until fragrant, about 30 seconds. Stir in soy sauce (or tamari) and red pepper flakes (if using).
3. **Toss:** Add the steamed green beans to the skillet and toss to coat.
4. **Garnish:** Sprinkle with sesame seeds (if using) and serve immediately.

- Spice it up: If you tolerate spice, add more red pepper flakes or a pinch of cayenne pepper.
- Nutty alternative: Swap sesame oil for a different neutral oil and add a sprinkle of chopped walnuts or almonds for crunch.

APPROXIMATE NUTRITIONAL INFO (PER SERVING)

- Calories: 100
- Protein: 4g
- Fiber: 4g

ROASTED CAULIFLOWER STEAKS WITH LEMON & HERBS DE PROVENCE

Prep time: 10 minutes | **Cook time:** 30-35 minutes | **Serving size:** 2 | **Special considerations:** Vegan, gluten-free, low in calories, easily customizable | **Budget-friendly tip:** Cauliflower is a versatile and affordable vegetable. Buy a whole head and use the florets for other dishes.

Why It's a GERD-Friendly Winner

These hearty cauliflower steaks are a delicious and satisfying alternative to meat. Roasting brings out the natural sweetness of cauliflower, while the lemon juice and herbs de Provence add a bright, Provençal flavor. This dish is low in fat and calories, making it a great option for those watching their weight.

INGREDIENTS

- 1 large head cauliflower, cut into 1-inch thick "steaks"
- 2 tablespoons olive oil
- Juice of 1 lemon
- 1 teaspoon dried herbs de Provence
- Salt and pepper to taste

INSTRUCTIONS

1. **Preheat oven to 400°F (200°C).**
2. **Prepare cauliflower:** Place the cauliflower steaks on a baking sheet lined with parchment paper.
3. **Season:** Drizzle with olive oil and lemon juice. Sprinkle with herbs de Provence, salt, and pepper.
4. **Roast:** Bake for 20-25 minutes, then flip the steaks and bake for another 10-15 minutes, or until tender and golden brown.

TIPS

- Spice it up: Add a pinch of red pepper flakes for a bit of heat.
- Serve with a dip: Enjoy these cauliflower steaks with a dollop of hummus or a drizzle of tahini sauce.

APPROXIMATE NUTRITIONAL INFO (PER SERVING)

- Calories: 200
- Protein: 5g
- Fiber: 10g

SAVORY MASHED SWEET POTATOES WITH CUMIN & CILANTRO

Prep time: 10 minutes | **Cook time:** 20-25 minutes | **Serving size:** 4 | **Special considerations:** Vegan, gluten-free, dairy-free, budget-friendly | **Budget-friendly tip:** Sweet potatoes are a very affordable and nutritious root vegetable. Buy them in bulk when they're in season.

Why It's a GERD-Friendly Winner

This flavorful twist on mashed sweet potatoes is a comforting and healthy side dish. Sweet potatoes are naturally sweet and packed with vitamins and fiber, while cumin adds warmth and depth. Cilantro provides a fresh, herbaceous note.

INGREDIENTS

- 2 large sweet potatoes, peeled and cubed
- 1 tablespoon olive oil
- ½ teaspoon cumin
- ¼ cup chopped fresh cilantro
- Salt and pepper to taste

INSTRUCTIONS

1. **Cook sweet potatoes:** Boil or steam the sweet potato cubes until very tender.
2. **Mash:** Drain the sweet potatoes and mash them with a potato masher or fork.
3. **Season:** Stir in olive oil, cumin, cilantro, salt, and pepper.

TIPS

- Spice it up: Add a pinch of cayenne pepper or chili powder for a little heat.

- Make it creamy: Stir in a dollop of non-dairy yogurt or a drizzle of olive oil for extra richness.

APPROXIMATE NUTRITIONAL INFO (PER SERVING)

- Calories: 150
- Fiber: 5g

TURMERIC ROASTED BROCCOLI

Prep time: 5 minutes | **Cook time:** 20-25 minutes | **Serving size:** 4 | Special considerations: Vegan, gluten-free | **Budget-friendly tip:** Broccoli is often on sale, and frozen broccoli florets can be a convenient and affordable alternative.

Why It's a GERD-Friendly Winner

This simple side dish is packed with flavor and anti-inflammatory benefits. Broccoli is a cruciferous vegetable that's high in fiber and vitamin C. Turmeric adds a vibrant color and its potent anti-inflammatory properties can help soothe the digestive system.

INGREDIENTS

- 1 head broccoli, cut into florets
- 1 tablespoon olive oil
- 1 teaspoon turmeric powder
- Salt and pepper to taste

INSTRUCTIONS

1. Preheat oven to 425°F (220°C).
2. Toss: In a large bowl, toss broccoli florets with olive oil, turmeric, salt, and pepper.
3. Roast: Spread the broccoli in a single layer on a baking sheet lined with parchment paper. Roast for 20-25 minutes, or until tender and lightly browned.

TIPS

- Spice it up: Add a pinch of red pepper flakes for a little heat.
- Garlic option: Toss the broccoli with minced garlic before roasting for extra flavor.
- Lemon zest: A sprinkle of lemon zest after roasting adds a bright and refreshing touch.

APPROXIMATE NUTRITIONAL INFO (PER SERVING)

- Calories: 100

- Fiber: 5g
- Vitamin C: 100% Daily Value

GINGER-PEACH SMOOTHIE BOWL

Prep time: 5 minutes | **Serving size:** 1 | **Special considerations:** Vegan, gluten-free, naturally sweet, easily customizable | **Budget-friendly tip:** Frozen peaches are a great way to enjoy the fruit year-round and often more affordable than fresh

Why It's a GERD-Friendly Winner

This vibrant and refreshing smoothie bowl is a delightful way to end your day on a light and healthy note. Frozen peaches and bananas offer natural sweetness and creamy texture, while ginger adds a warming, digestive-soothing touch. Spinach boosts the nutrient content, and a sprinkle of sliced almonds provides a satisfying crunch.

INGREDIENTS

- 1 cup frozen peaches
- ½ frozen banana
- 1 tablespoon grated fresh ginger
- ½ cup plain plant-based yogurt
- ½ cup packed spinach (fresh or frozen)
- Pinch of ground cinnamon
- Sliced almonds for topping

INSTRUCTIONS

1. Combine all ingredients (except almonds) in a blender.
2. Blend until smooth and creamy. If needed, add a splash of water or non-dairy milk for desired consistency.
3. Pour into a bowl and top with sliced almonds.

TIPS

- Sweetness adjustment: If you prefer a sweeter bowl, add a drizzle of honey or maple syrup.

- Topping ideas: Get creative with toppings like berries, granola, or a sprinkle of chia seeds.

- Make it a meal: Enjoy this bowl as a light dinner or a satisfying snack.

APPROXIMATE NUTRITIONAL INFO (PER SERVING)

- Calories: 250
- Protein: 8g
- Fiber: 6g
- Healthy Fats: 8g
- Vitamin C: 50% Daily Value

GRILLED SHRIMP & WATERMELON SKEWERS WITH BALSAMIC DRIZZLE

Prep time: 15 minutes | **Cook time:** 10-12 minutes | **Serving size:** 2 | **Special considerations:** Gluten-free, dairy-free, high in protein | **Budget-friendly tip:** Frozen shrimp can be a more affordable option than fresh

Why It's a GERD-Friendly Winner

These colorful skewers are a light and refreshing dinner option. Grilled shrimp provides lean protein, while watermelon adds natural sweetness and hydration. A touch of balsamic glaze adds a hint of acidity that complements the sweetness of the watermelon without being overwhelming.

INGREDIENTS

- 1 pound large shrimp, peeled and deveined
- 1 cup cubed watermelon
- 1 red bell pepper, cut into 1-inch pieces
- 1 tablespoon olive oil
- Salt and pepper to taste
- 1 tablespoon balsamic glaze
- Fresh basil leaves for garnish

INSTRUCTIONS

1. Soak wooden skewers in water for 30 minutes to prevent burning.
2. Thread shrimp, watermelon, and bell pepper pieces onto skewers.
3. Brush skewers with olive oil and season with salt and pepper.
4. Grill over medium heat for 2-3 minutes per side, or until shrimp is cooked through.
5. Drizzle with balsamic glaze and garnish with basil leaves

TIPS

- Marinate the shrimp: For extra flavor, marinate the shrimp in a mixture of olive oil, lemon juice, and herbs for 30 minutes before grilling.
- Vegetable variations: Feel free to substitute other GERD-friendly vegetables like zucchini or yellow squash.
- Serving suggestion: Serve these skewers with a side of brown rice or quinoa for a complete meal.

APPROXIMATE NUTRITIONAL INFO (PER SERVING)

- Calories: 300
- Protein: 25g
- Fiber: 3g
- Healthy Fats: 10g

AVOCADO & CUCUMBER SALAD WITH SESAME DRESSING

Prep time: 10 minutes | **Serving size:** 2 | **Special considerations:** Vegan, gluten-free, low in calories | **Budget-friendly tip:** Cucumbers are a very affordable vegetable, especially when in season.

Why It's a GERD-Friendly Winner

This simple and refreshing salad is perfect for a light dinner or a side dish. Avocado and cucumber are both hydrating and easy to digest, while the sesame dressing adds a nutty flavor without any spice or acidity.

INGREDIENTS

- Salad:
    - 2 avocados, sliced
    - 1 cucumber, sliced
    - Sesame seeds for garnish (optional)
- Sesame Dressing:
    - 2 tablespoons sesame oil
    - 1 tablespoon rice vinegar
    - 1 teaspoon honey (optional)
    - Pinch of salt

INSTRUCTIONS

1. Make dressing: In a small bowl, whisk together sesame oil, rice vinegar, honey (if using), and salt.
2. Assemble salad: Arrange avocado and cucumber slices on a plate.
3. Dress and serve: Drizzle the dressing over the salad and sprinkle with sesame seeds, if desired.

- Add protein: Top with grilled chicken or tofu for a more substantial meal.

- Make it a bowl: Serve the salad over a bed of brown rice or quinoa for a complete meal.

- Vary the dressing: Try using different types of vinegar, such as apple cider vinegar or white wine vinegar.

APPROXIMATE NUTRITIONAL INFO (PER SERVING)

- Calories: 300

- Healthy Fats: 25g

- Fiber: 8g

QUINOA-STUFFED PORTOBELLO MUSHROOMS

Prep time: 15 minutes | **Cook time:** 25-30 minutes | **Serving size: 2** | **Special considerations:** Vegetarian, gluten-free, high in protein | **Budget-friendly tip:** Look for portobello mushrooms on sale or buy them in bulk when they're in season

Why It's a GERD-Friendly Winner

These hearty stuffed mushrooms are a delicious and satisfying vegetarian meal. Portobello mushrooms provide a meaty texture and umami flavor, while quinoa adds protein and fiber. Spinach and walnuts offer additional nutrients, and a sprinkle of feta cheese adds a salty tang.

INGREDIENTS

- 2 large portobello mushrooms, stems removed and gills scraped out
- 1 cup cooked quinoa
- 1 cup chopped spinach
- ¼ cup chopped walnuts
- 2 tablespoons crumbled feta cheese
- 1 tablespoon olive oil
- Salt and pepper to taste

INSTRUCTIONS

1. **Preheat oven to 375°F (190°C).**
2. **Prepare mushrooms:** Brush the mushroom caps with olive oil and season with salt and pepper.
3. **Make filling:** In a bowl, combine quinoa, spinach, walnuts, feta, salt, and pepper.
4. **Stuff mushrooms:** Fill each mushroom cap with the quinoa mixture.

5. **Bake:** Place the stuffed mushrooms on a baking sheet and bake for 25-30 minutes, or until the mushrooms are tender and the filling is heated through.

TIPS

- Cheese variation: If you're avoiding dairy, omit the feta cheese or use a dairy-free alternative like vegan cheese or nutritional yeast.
- Make it ahead: The filling can be prepared in advance and refrigerated. Stuff the mushrooms just before baking.
- Serving suggestion: Serve these stuffed mushrooms with a side salad or a cup of GERD-friendly soup for a complete meal.

APPROXIMATE NUTRITIONAL INFO (PER SERVING)

- Calories: 350
- Protein: 15g
- Fiber: 10g
- Healthy Fats: 20g

SAVORY OATMEAL BOWL WITH CARAMELIZED ONIONS, MUSHROOMS & POACHED EGG

Prep time: 10 minutes | **Cook time:** 20 minutes | **Serving size**: 1 | **Special considerations:** Gluten-free (if using certified gluten-free oats), vegetarian, easily customizable | **Budget-friendly tip:** Oats are a pantry staple and can be purchased in bulk to save money. Choose mushrooms that are in season for the best value.

Why It's a GERD-Friendly Winner

This elevated take on oatmeal is surprisingly satisfying and gentle on digestion. Creamy oats provide a soothing base, while caramelized onions and mushrooms add savory depth and umami. A poached egg brings richness and protein, while chives provide a fresh, delicate onion flavor.

INGREDIENTS

- ½ cup rolled oats
- 1 cup low-sodium vegetable broth
- 1 tablespoon olive oil, divided
- 1 small onion, thinly sliced
- 4 ounces mushrooms (cremini, white button, or your choice), sliced
- 1 large egg
- 1 tablespoon chopped fresh chives
- Salt and pepper to taste
- Optional: A drizzle of balsamic glaze for a touch of sweetness

INSTRUCTIONS

1. **Cook oatmeal:** In a small saucepan, combine oats and vegetable broth. Bring to a simmer over medium heat, then reduce heat to low and cook for 5-7 minutes, or until the oats are tender and the liquid is absorbed.

2. **Caramelize onions:** While the oats are cooking, heat ½ tablespoon olive oil in a skillet over medium-low heat. Add the onions and cook, stirring occasionally, until deeply caramelized and golden brown, about 15-20 minutes.

3. **Sauté mushrooms:** In a separate skillet, heat the remaining ½ tablespoon olive oil over medium heat. Add the mushrooms and cook until softened and lightly browned, about 5-7 minutes. Season with salt and pepper.

4. **Poach egg:** Fill a separate saucepan with 2-3 inches of water and bring to a simmer. Add a teaspoon of white vinegar (this helps the egg white hold together). Gently crack the egg into a small bowl and slide it into the simmering water. Cook for 3-4 minutes until the white is set but the yolk is still runny. Remove with a slotted spoon and drain on a paper towel.

5. **Assemble:** Divide the cooked oatmeal between bowls. Top with caramelized onions, sautéed mushrooms, a poached egg, and chopped chives. Season with salt and pepper to taste. Drizzle with balsamic glaze, if desired.

TIPS

- Spice it up (if tolerated): Add a pinch of red pepper flakes for a touch of heat.
- Make it vegan: Substitute the poached egg with a scrambled tofu or a plant-based egg alternative.
- Top it off: Try adding a sprinkle of chopped walnuts or toasted pumpkin seeds for extra crunch and flavor.

APPROXIMATE NUTRITIONAL INFO (PER SERVING)

- Calories: 350
- Protein: 15g
- Fiber: 8g
- Healthy Fats: 18g

SAVORY OATMEAL BOWL WITH MUSHROOMS, POACHED EGG, AND CHIVES

Prep time: 5 minutes | **Cook time:** 15 minutes | **Serving size:** 1 | **Special considerations:** Gluten-free (if using certified gluten-free oats), vegetarian, easily **customizable** | **Budget-friendly tip:** Oats are an incredibly affordable pantry staple.

Why It's a GERD-Friendly Winner

This savory twist on oatmeal provides a warm and comforting dinner that's easy on the stomach. Oats offer a soothing base of soluble fiber, known for absorbing excess stomach acid. Mushrooms contribute umami flavor and essential nutrients, while the poached egg adds a boost of protein. Chives provide a subtle oniony flavor without being overly pungent.

INGREDIENTS

- ½ cup rolled oats

- 1 cup low-sodium vegetable broth

- ½ cup sliced mushrooms (cremini, white button, or your choice)

- 1 tablespoon olive oil

- 1 large egg

- 1 tablespoon chopped fresh chives

- Salt and pepper to taste

INSTRUCTIONS

1. **Cook oatmeal:** In a small saucepan, combine oats and vegetable broth. Bring to a simmer over medium heat, then reduce heat to low and cook for 5-7 minutes, or until the oats are tender and the liquid is absorbed.

2. **Sauté mushrooms:** While the oats are cooking, heat olive oil in a small skillet over medium heat. Add mushrooms and cook until softened and lightly browned, about 5-7 minutes. Season with salt and pepper.

3. **Poach egg:** Fill a separate saucepan with 2-3 inches of water and bring to a simmer. Add a teaspoon of vinegar (this helps the egg white hold together). Gently crack the egg into a small bowl and slide it into the simmering water. Cook for 3-4 minutes until the white is set but the yolk is still runny. Remove with a slotted spoon and drain on a paper towel.

4. **Assemble:** Divide the cooked oatmeal between bowls. Top with sautéed mushrooms, a poached egg, and chopped chives. Season with salt and pepper to taste.

TIPS

- Spice it up (if tolerated): Add a pinch of red pepper flakes for a touch of heat.
- Greens: Stir in a handful of spinach or kale at the end of cooking for added nutrients.
- Make it vegan: Substitute the poached egg with a scrambled tofu or a plant-based egg alternative.

APPROXIMATE NUTRITIONAL INFO (PER SERVING)

- Calories: 280
- Protein: 14g
- Fiber: 7g
- Healthy Fats: 12g

SNACKS & DESSERTS: SOOTHING SWEETNESS FOR GERD
TROPICAL GREEN MACHINE SMOOTHIE

Prep time: 5 minutes | **Serving size:** 1 | **Special considerations:** Vegan, gluten-free, naturally sweet, easily customizable | **Budget-friendly tip:** Buy frozen mango chunks in bulk to save money and have them on hand for smoothies year-round.

Why It's a GERD-Friendly Winner

This vibrant smoothie is packed with alkaline fruits and veggies that help soothe and neutralize stomach acid. Mango and avocado offer a creamy texture and healthy fats, while spinach provides a boost of vitamins and minerals. A touch of turmeric adds anti-inflammatory benefits, and a squeeze of lime brightens the flavors.

INGREDIENTS

- 1 cup frozen mango chunks
- ½ avocado, peeled and pitted
- 1 cup packed spinach (fresh or frozen)
- 1 cup unsweetened coconut milk (or your preferred non-dairy milk)
- ¼ teaspoon ground turmeric
- Juice of ½ lime

INSTRUCTIONS

1. Combine all ingredients in a blender.
2. Blend until smooth and creamy. If needed, add more coconut milk for desired consistency.
3. Pour into a glass and enjoy!

TIPS

- Adjust sweetness: If you prefer a sweeter smoothie, add a drizzle of honey or maple syrup.

- Make it tropical: Top with unsweetened coconut flakes or a few chunks of fresh pineapple.

- Boost the greens: Add a handful of kale or other leafy greens for extra nutrients.

APPROXIMATE NUTRITIONAL INFO (PER SERVING)

- Calories: 350
- Protein: 7g
- Fiber: 12g
- Healthy Fats: 20g
- Vitamin C: 80% Daily Value

CREAMY MELON REFRESHER SMOOTHIE

Prep time: 5 minutes | **Serving size:** 1 | **Special considerations:** Vegan, gluten-free, naturally sweet | **Budget-friendly tip:** Buy melons when they are in season for the best flavor and price.

Why It's a GERD-Friendly Winner

This smoothie is a hydrating and refreshing treat, perfect for a hot day or as a soothing snack. Cantaloupe or honeydew melon provide natural sweetness and hydration, while banana adds creaminess and potassium. A touch of ginger aids digestion, and chia seeds offer fiber and omega-3 fatty acids.

INGREDIENTS

- 1 cup frozen cantaloupe or honeydew melon chunks
- ½ frozen banana
- ½ cup plain plant-based yogurt
- ½ teaspoon grated fresh ginger
- 1 tablespoon chia seeds

INSTRUCTIONS

1. Combine all ingredients in a blender.
2. Blend until smooth and creamy. If needed, add a splash of water or non-dairy milk for desired consistency.
3. Pour into a glass and enjoy!

TIPS

- Add more greens: For extra nutrients, add a handful of spinach or kale.
- Make it minty: Toss in a few fresh mint leaves for a refreshing twist.
- Experiment with melon varieties: Try different types of melon for a variety of flavors.

APPROXIMATE NUTRITIONAL INFO (PER SERVING)

- Calories: 250
- Protein: 6g
- Fiber: 8g

BLUEBERRY BANANA BLAST SMOOTHIE

Prep time: 5 minutes | **Serving size:** 1 | **Special considerations:** Vegan, gluten-free (if using certified gluten-free oats), budget-friendly | **Budget-friendly tip:** Buy frozen blueberries in bulk to save money and have them on hand for smoothies.

Why It's a GERD-Friendly Winner

This classic smoothie combination is a crowd-pleaser for good reason. Blueberries and bananas are both low in acid and high in fiber, making them gentle on the stomach. The rolled oats add extra fiber and create a creamy texture, while almond milk provides a dose of healthy fats.

INGREDIENTS

- 1 cup frozen blueberries
- ½ frozen banana
- ¼ cup rolled oats
- 1 cup unsweetened almond milk (or your preferred milk)
- ½ teaspoon ground cinnamon
- 1 teaspoon honey or maple syrup (optional)

INSTRUCTIONS

1. Combine all ingredients in a blender.
2. Blend until smooth and creamy. If needed, add more milk for desired consistency.
3. Pour into a glass and enjoy!

- Add protein: For a more filling smoothie, add a scoop of protein powder or a tablespoon of nut butter.
- Make it green: Toss in a handful of spinach or kale for extra nutrients.
- Enjoy it warm: For a comforting twist, gently heat the smoothie in a saucepan before serving.

APPROXIMATE NUTRITIONAL INFO (PER SERVING)

- Calories: 300
- Protein: 8g
- Fiber: 10g
- Healthy Fats: 10g

PEANUT BUTTER BANANA POPSICLES

Prep time: 5 minutes | **Freeze time:** 4-6 hours | **Serving size:** 4 popsicles | **Special considerations:** Vegan, gluten-free, nut-free option (use sunflower seed butter instead of peanut butter)

Why It's a GERD-Friendly Winner

These creamy and satisfying popsicles are a healthy alternative to sugary frozen treats. Bananas are naturally sweet and low in acid, while peanut butter adds protein and healthy fats.

INGREDIENTS

- 2 ripe bananas
- ¼ cup creamy peanut butter (or sunflower seed butter)
- ½ cup unsweetened almond milk (or your preferred milk)

INSTRUCTIONS

1. Combine all ingredients in a blender and blend until smooth.
2. Pour the mixture into popsicle molds.
3. Freeze for 4-6 hours, or until solid.

TIPS

- Add chocolate: Drizzle melted dark chocolate (in moderation) over the popsicles before freezing for a decadent touch.
- Make it fun: Add sprinkles or chopped nuts to the popsicles before freezing.
- Enjoy as a snack or dessert: These popsicles are a refreshing treat for any time of day.

APPROXIMATE NUTRITIONAL INFO (PER SERVING)

- Calories: 150

- Protein: 5g
- Healthy Fats: 8g

GINGER PEACH NICE CREAM

Prep time: 5 minutes (plus freezing time for fruit) | **Serving size:** 2 | **Special considerations:** Vegan, gluten-free, naturally sweet

Why It's a GERD-Friendly Winner

This simple yet delicious frozen treat is made with just three ingredients. Peaches and bananas are naturally sweet and low in acid, while ginger adds a warming spice and aids digestion.

INGREDIENTS

- 2 cups frozen peaches
- 1 frozen banana
- 1 tablespoon grated fresh ginger

INSTRUCTIONS

1. Combine all ingredients in a food processor.
2. Process until smooth and creamy, scraping down the sides as needed.
3. Serve immediately as soft serve, or freeze for a firmer texture.

TIPS

- Add creaminess: For a richer texture, add a splash of coconut milk or almond milk.
- Spice it up: Add a pinch of cinnamon or nutmeg for extra warmth.
- Make it a parfait: Layer the nice cream with granola and berries for a more substantial snack.

APPROXIMATE NUTRITIONAL INFO (PER SERVING)

- Calories: 100
- Fiber: 3g

WATERMELON SKEWERS WITH FETA & MINT

Prep time: 5 minutes | **Serving size:** 2 skewers | **Special considerations:** Vegetarian, gluten-free, naturally sweet, low in calories | **Budget-friendly tip:** Watermelon is most affordable when in season. Feta can be purchased in blocks and crumbled to save money.

Why It's a GERD-Friendly Winner

These colorful skewers are a refreshing and satisfying snack. Watermelon is hydrating and alkaline, while feta adds a salty tang and mint offers a cooling touch. The combination of sweet and savory flavors makes this snack irresistible.

INGREDIENTS

- 2 cups cubed watermelon
- ¼ cup crumbled feta cheese
- 10-12 fresh mint leaves
- 4 wooden skewers

INSTRUCTIONS

1. Thread watermelon, feta, and mint leaves onto skewers.
2. Serve immediately or chill for a few minutes.

TIPS

- Get creative with skewers: Add other GERD-friendly fruits like honeydew melon or strawberries.
- Dairy-free option: Omit the feta cheese or use a dairy-free alternative.

APPROXIMATE NUTRITIONAL INFO (PER SERVING)

- Calories: 75
- Protein: 2g
- Fiber: 1g

CUCUMBER SLICES WITH HUMMUS & HERBS

Prep time: 5 minutes | **Serving size:** 1 | **Special considerations:** Vegan, gluten-free, high in fiber, customizable | **Budget-friendly tip:** Hummus is a versatile and affordable ingredient. You can easily make your own or buy it pre-made.

Why It's a GERD-Friendly Winner

This simple yet satisfying snack is packed with flavor and nutrients. Cucumbers are hydrating and alkaline, while hummus provides protein and fiber. The fresh herbs add a bright and aromatic touch.

INGREDIENTS

- 1 cucumber, sliced
- ¼ cup hummus (plain or flavored)
- Chopped fresh dill or parsley

INSTRUCTIONS

1. Spread hummus on cucumber slices.
2. Top with chopped herbs.

TIPS

- Variety is key: Try different hummus flavors and herbs to keep things interesting.
- Make it a meal: Pair with a side of whole-wheat crackers or pita bread for a more substantial snack.

APPROXIMATE NUTRITIONAL INFO (PER SERVING)

- Calories: 150
- Protein: 5g
- Fiber: 6g

BANANA & WALNUT BITES

Prep time: 5 minutes | **Serving size:** 1 | **Special considerations:** Vegan, gluten-free, nut-free option (use sunflower seed butter instead of nut butter)

Why It's a GERD-Friendly Winner

These bite-sized snacks are a delicious and nutritious way to satisfy your sweet tooth. Bananas are naturally sweet and gentle on the stomach, while walnuts provide protein, fiber, and healthy fats.

INGREDIENTS

- 1 banana, sliced
- 2 tablespoons nut butter (almond butter, cashew butter, etc.)
- 2 tablespoons chopped walnuts

INSTRUCTIONS

1. Spread nut butter on banana slices.
2. Top with chopped walnuts.

TIPS

- Change up the nut butter: Use your favorite variety, or try sunflower seed butter for a nut-free option.
- Add chocolate: Drizzle with melted dark chocolate (in moderation) for a decadent twist.

APPROXIMATE NUTRITIONAL INFO (PER SERVING)

- Calories: 200
- Protein: 6g
- Fiber: 4g
- Healthy Fats: 12g

FROZEN GRAPES

Prep time: 5 minutes | **Freeze time:** 2-3 hours | **Serving size:** 1 cup | **Special considerations:** Vegan, gluten-free, naturally sweet

Why It's a GERD-Friendly Winner

This simple snack is surprisingly refreshing and satisfying. Grapes are naturally sweet and low in acid, making them a great choice for people with GERD. Freezing them adds a fun twist and makes them even more enjoyable on a hot day.

INGREDIENTS

- 1 cup grapes, washed and dried

INSTRUCTIONS

1. Spread the grapes on a baking sheet lined with parchment paper.
2. Freeze for 2-3 hours, or until solid.

TIPS

- Choose your grapes: Red, green, or black grapes all work well for this recipe.
- Enjoy as a snack or dessert: These frozen grapes are a perfect way to cool down and satisfy your sweet cravings.

APPROXIMATE NUTRITIONAL INFO (PER SERVING)

- Calories: 60
- Fiber: 1g

ROASTED SWEET POTATO ROUNDS

Prep time: 10 minutes | **Cook time:** 20-25 minutes | **Serving size:** 2 | **Special considerations:** Vegan, gluten-free | **Budget-friendly tip:** Sweet potatoes are a very affordable and nutritious root vegetable.

Why It's a GERD-Friendly Winner

These crispy sweet potato rounds are a healthy and flavorful alternative to chips. Sweet potatoes are packed with nutrients and fiber, and roasting them brings out their natural sweetness. The cinnamon adds a touch of warmth without being irritating.

INGREDIENTS

- 1 large sweet potato, thinly sliced
- 1 tablespoon olive oil
- ½ teaspoon ground cinnamon
- Salt to taste

INSTRUCTIONS

1. **Preheat oven to 400°F (200°C).**
2. **Toss:** In a bowl, toss sweet potato slices with olive oil, cinnamon, and salt.
3. **Roast:** Spread the slices in a single layer on a baking sheet lined with parchment paper. Roast for 20-25 minutes, flipping halfway through, until tender and golden brown.

TIPS

- Spice it up: Add a pinch of cayenne pepper for a subtle kick of heat.
- Dip it: Enjoy with a side of hummus or guacamole.

APPROXIMATE NUTRITIONAL INFO (PER SERVING)

- Calories: 150
- Fiber: 4g

CHAPTER 5

BEYOND THE PLATE: NAVIGATING THE GERD JOURNEY WITH CONFIDENCE

Congratulations! You've made it this far, diving into the world of GERD-friendly eating and discovering delicious recipes that nourish your body and soul. But the journey doesn't end here. In this chapter, we'll explore how to go beyond the plate and equip you with the knowledge and tools to thrive with GERD in the long run.

When to Call in the Cavalry: Signs You Need Medical Help

While diet and lifestyle changes can work wonders for managing GERD, sometimes your body needs a little extra support. It's crucial to recognize the signs that your reflux might be more than just a minor inconvenience. If you experience any of the following, don't hesitate to talk to your doctor:

- **Difficulty or Painful Swallowing:** This could indicate that acid reflux has caused inflammation or damage to your esophagus.
- **Unexplained Weight Loss:** While some weight loss is a positive side effect of a healthier diet, sudden or unexplained weight loss can be a red flag for a more serious underlying issue.
- **Anemia:** Acid reflux can sometimes lead to bleeding in the esophagus, which can result in anemia (low red blood cell count). Symptoms of anemia include fatigue, weakness, and pale skin.
- **Persistent Vomiting or Nausea:** Occasional nausea is common with GERD, but persistent vomiting or nausea could signal a complication.
- **Black or Bloody Stools:** This could be a sign of bleeding in your digestive tract, which requires immediate medical attention.

If you notice any of these symptoms, don't panic. Most GERD complications can be effectively managed with medication and lifestyle modifications. But early detection is key, so don't hesitate to seek help if something doesn't feel right.

The Medication Maze: Finding What Works for You

Sometimes, lifestyle changes alone aren't enough to tame GERD. That's where medications come in. They can be a powerful tool for reducing acid production, strengthening your lower esophageal sphincter, and healing any damage to your esophagus. But remember, it's important to work closely with your doctor to find the right medication and dosage for you.

There are several types of medications commonly used to treat GERD, including:

- **Antacids:** These over-the-counter medications work by neutralizing stomach acid. They can provide quick relief from heartburn, but they don't address the underlying cause of GERD.
- **H2 Blockers:** These medications reduce acid production in your stomach. They can provide longer relief than antacids, but they may not be strong enough for everyone.
- **Proton Pump Inhibitors (PPIs):** PPIs are the most powerful medications for reducing stomach acid. They work by blocking the pumps that produce acid in your stomach. PPIs can be very effective for healing esophageal damage and managing severe GERD symptoms.

Your doctor will help you determine which medication is right for you based on the severity of your symptoms, your medical history, and other factors. It's important to follow your doctor's instructions carefully and to be aware of any potential side effects of the medication you're taking.

The Long Game: Building a Sustainable GERD-Friendly Lifestyle

Managing GERD isn't a sprint; it's a marathon. It's about making sustainable changes to your diet and lifestyle that you can stick with for the long haul. Here are a few tips for long-term success:

- **Keep a food diary:** Track what you eat and how you feel to identify your personal trigger foods.

- **Eat regular meals:** Avoid skipping meals or going too long without eating, as this can trigger acid production.
- **Practice mindful eating:** Slow down and savor your food. This can help you eat less and reduce the risk of overeating, which can worsen reflux symptoms.
- **Manage stress:** Find healthy ways to manage stress, such as exercise, meditation, or spending time in nature.
- **Prioritize sleep:** Aim for 7-8 hours of quality sleep each night.
- **Maintain a healthy weight:** If you're overweight or obese, losing even a small amount of weight can significantly improve your GERD symptoms.
- **Stay active:** Regular physical activity can help improve digestion and reduce stress.
- **Avoid smoking and excessive alcohol:** These habits can weaken your LES and irritate your esophagus.

You're in Control

Remember, you're not alone in this journey. Millions of people live with GERD, and there are countless resources and support systems available to help you thrive. This cookbook is just one tool in your arsenal. By making informed choices about your diet, lifestyle, and medication, you can take control of your health and enjoy a life free from the limitations of GERD.

This isn't the end of the book; it's just the beginning of a new chapter in your life. A chapter filled with delicious food, good health, and the freedom to enjoy every bite.

CHAPTER 6

60 DAYS MEAL PLAN

Week 1

Day	Breakfast	Lunch	Dinner	Snack
1	Banana Berry Blast Smoothie	Mediterranean Quinoa Bowl	Ginger-Glazed Salmon with Roasted Vegetables	Cucumber Slices with Hummus & Herbs
2	Apple Spice Delight Oatmeal	Grilled Chicken & Pineapple-Free Salsa Wrap	Roasted Butternut Squash & Lentil Soup	Watermelon Skewers with Feta & Mint
3	Savory Sunshine Bowl	Herbed Lentil & Cucumber Salad	Lemony Herb Chicken with Asparagus & Zucchini	Frozen Grapes
4	Blueberry Bliss Oatmeal	Watermelon, Feta & Mint Salad	Tofu Scramble with Spinach & Mushrooms	Banana & Walnut Bites
5	Tropical Green Dream Smoothie	Spinach & Avocado Salad	Stuffed Bell Peppers	Roasted Sweet Potato Rounds
6	Creamy Ginger Peach Smoothie	Hummus & Veggie Pinwheels	Sweet Potato Black Bean Burgers	
7	Spinach & Feta Scramble with Toast	Lentil & Sauerkraut Wrap	Herbed Quinoa & White Bean Salad	

Day	Breakfast	Lunch	Dinner	Snack
8	Veggie-Packed Frittata Bites	Mediterranean Quinoa Bowl	Roasted Garlic & Cauliflower Soup	Banana & Walnut Bites
9	Turmeric Scramble with Avocado	Sesame-Crusted Chicken & Kale Salad	Chicken & Veggie Coconut Curry	Cucumber Slices with Hummus & Herbs
10	Banana Buckwheat Pancakes	Herbed Lentil & Cucumber Salad	Shrimp & Avocado Quinoa Bowls	Frozen Grapes
11	Sweet Potato Hash	Watermelon, Feta & Mint Salad	Herb-Crusted Salmon w/ Asparagus & Beans	Roasted Sweet Potato Rounds
12	Avocado Toast Deluxe	Spinach & Avocado Salad	Tofu Scramble w/ Spinach & Mushrooms	
13	Melon & Mint Salad	Hummus & Veggie Pinwheels	Stuffed Bell Peppers	
14	Simple Green Goodness with Bacon	Lentil & Sauerkraut Wrap	Sweet Potato Black Bean Burgers on Lettuce	

Week 3

Day	Breakfast	Lunch	Dinner	Snack
15	Banana Berry Blast Smoothie	Mediterranean Quinoa Bowl	Lemony Herb Chicken with Asparagus & Zucchini	Frozen Grapes
16	Apple Spice Delight Oatmeal	Grilled Chicken & Pineapple-Free Salsa Wrap	Roasted Butternut Squash & Lentil Soup	Cucumber Slices with Hummus & Herbs
17	Savory Sunshine Bowl	Herbed Lentil & Cucumber Salad	Tofu Scramble with Spinach & Mushrooms	Watermelon Skewers with Feta & Mint
18	Blueberry Bliss Oatmeal	Watermelon, Feta & Mint Salad	Stuffed Bell Peppers	Banana & Walnut Bites
19	Tropical Green Dream Smoothie	Spinach & Avocado Salad	Sweet Potato Black Bean Burgers	Roasted Sweet Potato Rounds
20	Creamy Ginger Peach Smoothie	Hummus & Veggie Pinwheels	Herb-Crusted Salmon w/ Asparagus & Beans	
21	Spinach & Feta Scramble with Toast	Lentil & Sauerkraut Wrap	Herbed Quinoa & White Bean Salad	

Week 4

Day	Breakfast	Lunch	Dinner	Snack
22	Veggie-Packed Frittata Bites	Mediterranean Quinoa Bowl	Roasted Garlic & Cauliflower Soup	Cucumber Slices with Hummus & Herbs
23	Turmeric Scramble with Avocado	Sesame-Crusted Chicken & Kale Salad	Chicken & Veggie Coconut Curry	Banana & Walnut Bites
24	Banana Buckwheat Pancakes	Herbed Lentil & Cucumber Salad	Shrimp & Avocado Quinoa Bowls	Roasted Sweet Potato Rounds
25	Sweet Potato Hash	Watermelon, Feta & Mint Salad	Mediterranean Baked Fish	Frozen Grapes
26	Avocado Toast Deluxe	Spinach & Avocado Salad	Tofu Scramble w/ Spinach & Mushrooms	
27	Melon & Mint Salad	Hummus & Veggie Pinwheels	Stuffed Bell Peppers	
28	Simple Green Goodness with Bacon	Lentil & Sauerkraut Wrap	Sweet Potato Black Bean Burgers on Lettuce	

Week 5

Day	Breakfast	Lunch	Dinner	Snack
29	Banana Buckwheat Pancakes	Roasted Garlic & Cauliflower Soup	Shrimp & Avocado Quinoa Bowls	Cucumber Slices with Hummus & Herbs
30	Savory Oatmeal Bowl	Hummus & Veggie Pinwheels	Ginger-Glazed Salmon with Roasted Vegetables	Frozen Grapes
31	Blueberry Bliss Oatmeal	Grilled Chicken & Pineapple-Free Salsa Wrap	Roasted Butternut Squash & Lentil Soup	Watermelon Skewers with Feta & Mint
32	Tropical Green Dream Smoothie	Lentil & Sauerkraut Wrap	Lemony Herb Chicken with Asparagus & Zucchini	Banana & Walnut Bites
33	Creamy Ginger Peach Smoothie	Herb-Crusted Salmon w/ Asparagus & Beans	Tofu Scramble with Spinach & Mushrooms	Roasted Sweet Potato Rounds
34	Spinach & Feta Scramble with Toast	Chicken & Quinoa Stuffed Peppers	Herbed Quinoa & White Bean Salad	
35	Veggie-Packed Frittata Bites	Mediterranean Quinoa Bowl	Sweet Potato Black Bean Burgers on Lettuce	

Day	Breakfast	Lunch	Dinner	Snack
36	Turmeric Scramble with Avocado	Roasted Garlic & Cauliflower Soup	Chicken & Veggie Coconut Curry	Banana & Walnut Bites
37	Sweet Potato Hash	Hummus & Veggie Pinwheels	Shrimp & Avocado Quinoa Bowls	Roasted Sweet Potato Rounds
38	Avocado Toast Deluxe	Grilled Chicken & Pineapple-Free Salsa Wrap	Mediterranean Baked Fish	Frozen Grapes
39	Melon & Mint Salad	Lentil & Sauerkraut Wrap	Tofu Scramble w/ Spinach & Mushrooms	
40	Simple Green Goodness with Bacon	Herb-Crusted Salmon w/ Asparagus & Beans	Stuffed Bell Peppers	
41	Banana Berry Blast Smoothie	Chicken & Quinoa Stuffed Peppers	Sweet Potato Black Bean Burgers	
42	Apple Spice Delight Oatmeal	Mediterranean Quinoa Bowl	Herbed Quinoa & White Bean Salad	

Week 7

Day	Breakfast	Lunch	Dinner	Snack
43	Savory Sunshine Bowl	Roasted Garlic & Cauliflower Soup	Lemony Herb Chicken & Veggies	Frozen Grapes
44	Blueberry Bliss Oatmeal	Hummus & Veggie Pinwheels	Sweet Potato Black Bean Burgers	Banana & Walnut Bites
45	Tropical Green Dream Smoothie	Grilled Chicken & Pineapple-Free Salsa Wrap	Herb-Crusted Salmon & Sides	Roasted Sweet Potato Rounds
46	Creamy Ginger Peach Smoothie	Lentil & Sauerkraut Wrap	Mediterranean Baked Fish	
47	Spinach & Feta Scramble with Toast	Chicken & Quinoa Stuffed Peppers	Tofu Scramble & Roasted Potatoes	
48	Veggie-Packed Frittata Bites	Mediterranean Quinoa Bowl	Stuffed Bell Peppers	
49	Turmeric Scramble with Avocado	Sesame-Crusted Chicken & Kale Salad	Herbed Quinoa & White Bean Salad	

Week 8

Day	Breakfast	Lunch	Dinner	Snack
50	Sweet Potato Hash	Herbed Lentil & Cucumber Salad	Roasted Garlic & Cauliflower Soup	Cucumber Slices with Hummus & Herbs
51	Avocado Toast Deluxe	Watermelon, Feta & Mint Salad	Ginger-Glazed Salmon with Roasted Vegetables	Banana & Walnut Bites
52	Melon & Mint Salad	Spinach & Avocado Salad	Chicken & Veggie Coconut Curry	Roasted Sweet Potato Rounds
53	Simple Green Goodness with Bacon	Hummus & Veggie Pinwheels	Shrimp & Avocado Quinoa Bowls	Frozen Grapes
54	Banana Buckwheat Pancakes	Grilled Chicken & Pineapple-Free Salsa Wrap	Mediterranean Baked Fish	
55	Savory Oatmeal Bowl	Lentil & Sauerkraut Wrap	Tofu Scramble with Spinach & Mushrooms	
56	Blueberry Bliss Oatmeal	Herb-Crusted Salmon w/ Asparagus & Beans	Sweet Potato Black Bean Burgers on Lettuce	

Recipe Substitutions and Tips for Creating Your Own GERD Meal Plan:

One of the greatest benefits of a GERD-friendly diet is its flexibility. While the 60-day meal plan offers a structured guide, you're not locked into it. Feel free to swap recipes, adjust portion sizes, and experiment with different ingredients to suit your preferences and needs.

Here are some key tips for creating your own GERD meal plan and making successful substitutions:

1. Understand Your Triggers:
    - Keep a food diary: Track what you eat and any symptoms you experience to identify your personal trigger foods.
    - Common triggers: Fatty foods, acidic foods (citrus, tomatoes), spicy foods, chocolate, peppermint, alcohol, caffeine, and carbonated beverages.
    - Individual differences: Not everyone reacts the same way to every food. Pay attention to your body's unique responses.

2. Prioritize GERD-Friendly Foods:
    - Focus on lean proteins, fruits, vegetables, whole grains, and healthy fats (like those found in avocados, nuts, and olive oil).
    - Choose low-acid fruits like berries, melons, and bananas.
    - Opt for cooked vegetables over raw, as they are often easier to digest.
    - Limit or avoid highly processed foods, sugary drinks, and fried foods.

3. Make Smart Substitutions:
    - Protein: Swap chicken for fish, turkey, or tofu. Replace red meat with lentils, beans, or eggs (just the whites).
    - Grains: Use brown rice instead of white rice, quinoa instead of couscous, or gluten-free options if needed.

- Vegetables: Choose low-acid options like broccoli, asparagus, cauliflower, zucchini, leafy greens, and cucumbers.
  - Fats: Opt for olive oil, avocado oil, or nut butters instead of butter or high-fat dairy.
  - Dairy: If dairy is a trigger, replace cow's milk with almond milk, oat milk, or other plant-based alternatives.
  - Spices: Use herbs like dill, parsley, and cilantro for flavor instead of spicy peppers or chilies.

4. Ensure a Balanced Diet:
  - Include a variety of foods from all food groups to ensure you're getting all the essential nutrients your body needs.
  - Aim for a balance of protein, healthy fats, and carbohydrates in each meal.
  - Don't forget about fiber! Incorporate plenty of fruits, vegetables, and whole grains into your diet.

5. Cooking Methods:
  - Opt for grilling, baking, roasting, or steaming over frying, as these methods are gentler on the digestive system.
  - Avoid adding extra fat to your cooking.

6. Portion Control:
  - Even healthy foods can trigger reflux if you eat too much at once. Be mindful of your portion sizes.
  - Try eating smaller, more frequent meals throughout the day instead of large meals.

7. Hydration:
  - Stay hydrated by drinking plenty of water throughout the day.
  - Herbal teas like chamomile and ginger can also be soothing for the digestive system.

8. Listen to Your Body:

- Pay attention to how you feel after eating certain foods. If something seems to trigger your symptoms, avoid it or try it in smaller amounts.
- Everyone is different, so what works for one person may not work for another. Experiment and find what works best for you.

A Balanced GERD-Friendly Diet: What to Aim For

A balanced diet for GERD focuses on nourishing your body while minimizing triggers. Here's what you should aim to include in your daily meals:

- Lean Protein:
  - Examples: Chicken breast, turkey, fish, seafood, egg whites, lentils, beans, tofu, tempeh
  - Why it's important: Protein helps build and repair tissues, keeps you feeling full, and supports a healthy metabolism.
  - Recipes: Ginger-Glazed Salmon, Lemony Herb Chicken, Shrimp & Avocado Quinoa Bowls, Tofu Scramble, Lentil & Sauerkraut Wrap
- Healthy Fats:
  - Examples: Avocados, nuts, seeds, olive oil, sesame oil
  - Why it's important: Healthy fats support cell growth, hormone production, and nutrient absorption. They also help you feel satisfied and can reduce inflammation.
  - Recipes: Avocado Toast Deluxe, Mediterranean Quinoa Bowl, Spinach & Avocado Salad, Roasted Garlic & Cauliflower Soup
- Complex Carbohydrates:

- Examples: Quinoa, brown rice, oats, whole-wheat bread, sweet potatoes, butternut squash, legumes
    - Why it's important: Complex carbohydrates provide sustained energy, fiber, and essential nutrients. They're digested more slowly than simple carbs, helping to prevent blood sugar spikes and crashes.
    - Recipes: Mediterranean Quinoa Bowl, Sweet Potato Hash, Curried Sweet Potato Soup, Banana Buckwheat Pancakes
- Fiber:
    - Examples: Fruits, vegetables, whole grains, legumes
    - Why it's important: Fiber aids digestion, promotes regular bowel movements, and helps absorb excess stomach acid.
    - Recipes: All salads, Roasted Vegetables, Hummus & Veggie Pinwheels
- Low-Acid Fruits:
    - Examples: Bananas, melons, berries, apples, pears
    - Why it's important: Low-acid fruits are less likely to trigger heartburn and reflux symptoms.
    - Recipes: Banana Berry Blast Smoothie, Creamy Melon Refresher Smoothie, Blueberry Banana Blast Smoothie
- Non-Starchy Vegetables:
    - Examples: Broccoli, cauliflower, asparagus, green beans, leafy greens, cucumbers
    - Why it's important: These vegetables are low in calories and high in nutrients, making them an important part of a GERD-friendly diet.
    - Recipes: Roasted Cauliflower Steaks, Garlic-Sesame Green Beans, Turmeric Roasted Broccoli

Sample Balanced Meal Plan for One Day:

- Breakfast: Oatmeal with Berries and Almond Milk

- Provides: Complex carbohydrates (oats), fiber (berries), healthy fats (almond milk)
- Lunch: Grilled Chicken Salad with Mixed Greens and Avocado
    - Provides: Lean protein (chicken), healthy fats (avocado), fiber (mixed greens)
- Dinner: Baked Salmon with Roasted Asparagus and Lemon-Dill Sauce
    - Provides: Lean protein (salmon), healthy fats (salmon and olive oil), fiber (asparagus)
- Snacks: Cucumber slices with hummus, berries
    - Provides: Protein and fiber (hummus), fiber and vitamins (berries)

Tips for Creating Your Own Balanced Meal Plan:

- Use the recipes in this book as a starting point: The recipes provided are already designed to be GERD-friendly and balanced, so feel free to use them as a base for your meal plan.
- Focus on whole, unprocessed foods: Choose foods that are as close to their natural state as possible, avoiding highly processed foods that are often high in unhealthy fats, sugar, and sodium.
- Read labels carefully: Pay attention to the ingredient list and nutrition facts panel to make informed choices.

CONCLUSION

SAVOR THE FLAVOR, RECLAIM YOUR LIFE

As you close this cookbook, I hope you feel a renewed sense of hope and excitement about food. Remember, managing GERD doesn't have to mean sacrificing flavor or enjoyment. It's about discovering new ways to nourish your body, embrace a variety of delicious ingredients, and create a sustainable, GERD-friendly lifestyle that truly works for you.

I promise you this: with knowledge, creativity, and a willingness to experiment, you can absolutely live a life filled with vibrant, satisfying meals that also support your digestive health. This cookbook is just the beginning of your culinary adventure. Let it be your guide as you explore new flavors, try different combinations, and discover your own personal GERD-friendly favorites.

Remember, food is meant to be enjoyed. It's a source of pleasure, connection, and nourishment. Don't let GERD rob you of that joy. With the tools and information you've gained from this book, you're equipped to take charge of your health and reclaim your love of food.

Go forth, cook with confidence, and savor every delicious bite!

A Special Note from the Author

Dear Reader,

Thank you for embarking on this culinary journey with me. This cookbook is a labor of love, born out of my passion for helping people like you rediscover the joy of eating while managing GERD.

I'd love to hear from you! Your feedback is invaluable to me. Did you enjoy the recipes? Were the tips and information helpful? Do you have any questions or suggestions for future editions?

Please feel free to share your thoughts and experiences with me. Your feedback will help me continue to create resources that empower and support you on your GERD journey.